A Short History of
Medical Ethics

A Short History of
MEDICAL ETHICS

ALBERT R. JONSEN

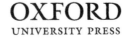

OXFORD
UNIVERSITY PRESS

OXFORD

UNIVERSITY PRESS

Oxford University Press, Inc., publishes works that further
Oxford University's objective of excellence
in research, scholarship, and education.

Oxford   New York
Auckland   Cape Town   Dar es Salaam   Hong Kong   Karachi
Kuala Lumpur   Madrid   Melbourne   Mexico City   Nairobi
New Delhi   Shanghai   Taipei   Toronto

With offices in
Argentina   Austria   Brazil   Chile   Czech Republic   France   Greece
Guatemala   Hungary   Italy   Japan   Poland   Portugal   Singapore
South Korea   Switzerland   Thailand   Turkey   Ukraine   Vietnam

Copyright © 2000 by Oxford University Press, Inc.

Published by Oxford University Press, Inc.
198 Madison Avenue, New York, New York 10016

www.oup.com

First issued as an Oxford University Press paperback, 2008

Oxford is a registered trademark of Oxford University Press

Library of Congress Cataloguing-in-Publication Data
Jonsen, Albert R.
A short history of medical ethics / Albert R. Jonsen.
p.   cm.
Includes bibliographical references and index.
ISBN- 978-0-19-536984-7
1. Medical ethics–History   I. Title.
R724.J665 2000
174'.2'09-dc21   99-14646

Printed in the United States of America
on acid-free paper

Preface

Thirty years ago, when I first joined the faculty of a medical school, my title, Professor of Medical Ethics, was an unusual one, difficult to explain, particularly to senior physicians, who took the ethics of their profession for granted. They believed in simple rules, such as firm dedication and courtesy to one's patients, confidentiality, and the duty to provide free care for the poor. What need was there for a professor, particularly one who was not a physician, to teach these maxims? Examples set by revered teachers and colleagues certainly sufficed to convey the traditional ethics of the profession. These skeptics of my professorial status had a point: there was a long tradition of simple but stringent duties that rarely demanded close analysis. If there was a problem, it was the moral failure to observe these duties rather than the need to puzzle over their meaning.

But the skeptics were looking to the past. They did not see how strongly medicine's growing technical and scientific capabilities pressed on their duties as the tradition defined them. The dynamic of scientific investigation drew physicians into experiments with their patients that, on the surface at least, seemed to violate the old rule to do no harm. The power of life-sustaining technologies and the miracles of organ transplantation confounded settled understandings about when the moment of death occurred and how to care for the dying. Molecular genetics offered information about the risks of disease that had not yet appeared in signs and symptoms and discomfited the old rule of confidentiality. The practitioner's world had been surrounded by complex institutions for the financing and delivery of medical care, raising doubts about how the doctor's allegiance to patients could be reconciled with the interests of multiple parties. These and many other changes, in medicine and in cultural values, were pressuring the old tradition to make its assumptions clearer and to revise its settled values. For the last 30 years, that medical world has been roiled by constant debates about the ethical dimensions of caring for patients, introducing new technologies, and exploring promising, yet strange, scientific paths.

Now people say to me, "Oh, how interesting it must be to teach medical ethics! Did you see the story in yesterday's paper about . . . ?" The pressures that were pushing on the old tradition now break out into almost daily dramatic stories. Medical ethics, or its newer version, bioethics, is a matter of wide interest among the public and the profession. Yet, as the new medical ethics burgeons, the lines of the old tradition fade. Not that some of the stringent duties, such as the obligation to refrain from doing harm, have disappeared; rather, their origins and their place in the development of the medical profession are not well known. Since in many ways those traditional duties still stand as the background of the new, more analytic ethics of medicine, it seems worthwhile to review the evolution of the tradition of medical ethics.

Until recently, historians of medicine have paid little attention to medical ethics in other eras and cultures. Apart from a few famous essays exploring the ethics of Hippocratic medicine, vast eras were left unexplored. Original sources were difficult to find, and few scholars were dedicated to mining them. In recent years, as historians of medicine emphasized the social history of medicine, they discovered writings about medical ethics from many eras. A recent volume of essays on the history of medical ethics opened with the author's intention to "tackle the gap on the subject" that exists between the "oft cited 'origins' of medical ethics, the Hippocratic Oath and Thomas Percival's *Medical Ethics* of 1803." As the interest in bioethics has grown, so has the interest in the history of medical ethics. Today, several scholarly projects are delving into the social, cultural, and philosophical grounds of the traditional ethics of medicine.[1]

This is a history book written by one who never studied the formal methods of historical research and writing. Thus, it is likely to be marred by blunders that make scholarly historians shudder: unknowing neglect of sources of evidence that might expand or contradict the author's view, jumbling eras and cultures that should be distinguished, and, perhaps worst of all, giving generous, firm interpretations to tenuous and ambiguous evidence. In compensation for these faults of an amateur historian, the references to scholarly literature are more ample than might be usual in so small a book. Certainly, this book will be surpassed by more careful scholarly investigations, both in correctness and in amplitude. Yet, it will be some years before the current projects on the history of medicine produce a comprehensive corpus of studies. In the meantime, this short history can serve those who are curious about the history of medical ethics.

I acknowledge with gratitude the critical assessment of some genuine scholars: Professors Darrel Amundsen, James Whorton, Robert Baker, Patricia Ebrey, Frank Conlon, Zev Handel, and two masked readers who read the drafts at the invitation of Oxford University Press. The help of my research assistant, Ms. Kelly Edwards, and the editing by my wife, Mary Elizabeth, have been invaluable.

Seattle, Wash.   A.R.J.
January 1999

Contents

Introduction
The Long Tradition of Ethics in Medicine

The reader is about to embark on a short tour through the long tradition of moral discourse about medicine. Like most tours, this one stops at the most salient points of interest and sails rather quickly past the rich cultural background in which the indigenous medicine grew. This intellectual itinerary has its perils. It may, in the hope of finding themes, miss important differences. The very word *tradition*, when applied to discourse about morality in medicine, signals that peril. It may disguise the diversity of the discourse that takes place in varied centuries and cultures. Some scholars warn that no continuous stream flows from ancient to modern times.[1] Certainly, concepts and practices about virtue and rectitude, even when they share similar names over centuries, differ in meaning over the centuries and within the cultures that cultivate them. Athenian democracy is vastly different from American democracy, and though we might use the quaint word *magnanimous* to praise a generous benefactor, Aristotle's "magnanimous man" appears to us an arrogant snob. Despite this acknowledgment of cultural and temporal differences, the literature about medical ethics does seem to circle around certain common themes, recognizable even under distinct guises. Those themes can be discerned in the words of writers from many lands and times. Those words coalesce into a long tradition, even though their modern readers must recognize that, while the words can be translated from Greek or Latin or French or Chinese, the meanings often cling to the worlds in which they were written. Even with this caution about too easily transporting the themes from their home cultures into ours, there is, I believe, a long tradition of medical ethics in the civilizations of both East and West.

This history is also about a tradition of ethics. The word *ethics* carries a number of meanings, from the study of morality (Aristotle's *Ethics* is a book about "the knowledge of the Supreme Good which is of practical importance to the conduct of life")[2] to the behavior of persons who act in or out of accord with some standard, either of human excellence (the ethics of Mohandas Gandhi are admirable) or of conventional norms (the ethics of Congressman Sly flaunt the federal law on fundraising). When applied to professional behavior, the word *ethics* acquires yet other meanings: "much of what can be called 'ethics'," says a sociologist of medicine, "is designed to prevent 'unfair' internal competition . . . in the medical marketplace, at the same time that it presents an impeccable front of silence to the outside world."[3] This variety of meanings confuses the discussion of medical ethics: are we addressing the actual behavior of doctors, or the rules that doctors ought to follow in their relations with their patients and colleagues, or the deeper moral principles that should guide physicians, just as they should guide all persons? Is medical ethics a set of rules expressed in a written code promulgated by medical associations or is it a study of how the general principles of morality pertain to medical practice? Is it hardly ethics at all but instead a set of doctor-created conventions to preserve professional prestige and monopoly?

Despite the multifarious meanings of morality and ethics, it is possible to discover, in the writings of those who have reflected about the nature of the moral life, several consistent themes. From the time of Socrates on, these thinkers have reflected on the character or quality of the moral person, on the duties or obligations that constitute a moral life, and on the relationship between individuals and their community. For convenience, these three domains of ethics will be designated as *decorum, deontology*, and *politic ethics*. *Decorum*, a word Cicero used to describe outward behaviors that manifest inner virtue, comprises a variety of attitudes and actions, with names such as *politeness, courage, respectfulness*, and *resoluteness*. These qualities are often entitled *virtues* (or *vices*). *Deontology*, a modern word formed from the Greek word *deon*, meaning "duty" or "obligation," comprises the part of morality that is built around conceptions of what one ought to do and finds expression in rules and principles. Finally, *politic ethics* looks beyond the individual to the community within which individuals live their lives. The moral idea of justice invokes the moral dimension of this relationship. The rather unusual phrase *politic ethics* has been chosen for reasons that will become clear as we move through this history.

When one turns from moral philosophy to medical ethics, these three domains come into sight. They may not be explored at the depth that a philosopher's ruminations might reach, but, again and again, the medical life is seen as one in which certain persons, called physicians, have certain duties toward others, their patients. The physicians, in order to fulfill those duties properly, must display qualities of mind, will, and affections and behave in manifest ways related to those qualities. Finally, physicians not only care for the sick who are their patients; they play a part in a larger community and must serve its welfare. Thus, medical decorum, deontology, and politic ethics will be constant refrains as the long tradition is traced throughout history.

Through the tradition, these refrains will be repeated in remarkably similar tones but with considerable variety in emphasis. For example, the manners recommended in the decorum have great stability, even though they are described differently in the conventional prose of particular eras. Other elements of decorum, such as confidentiality or the medical secret, present since earliest times, are stressed differently in different cultures and even become integrated into the deontology. Elements of the deontology, such as rules against performing abortion or against deliberately taking life, rest on deep moral presuppositions that appear consistently but rather differently from one era and culture to another. The authors of the Hippocratic admonitions to refrain from performing abortion or assisting suicide certainly viewed the moral meaning of those rules quite differently than did the physicians of ten centuries later, who swore the Hippocratic Oath "as a Christian may swear it." Politic ethics, rarely mentioned in ancient medicine, grows in importance as medicine becomes a professional practice in commercial cultures. There is a long tradition, then, but caution is advised about distilling its complexity into a simple uniformity.

Much of the long tradition was created by physicians writing about how physicians ought to behave. However, medical morality is much wider. It includes the responses of other individuals and institutions to medical activities. Thus, the comments of poets and playwrights, the teachings of rabbis and popes, and the decrees of kings and councils will appear in these pages. These comments on medical morality may not fit neatly the schema of deontology, duty, and politic ethics, but they do shed light on the general conception of the links between medicine and morality.

A Short History of
Medical Ethics

1

Hellenic, Hellenistic, and Roman Medicine
Fifth Century BCE to Third Century CE

The ethics of medicine in Western culture has its roots in Hellenic, Hellenistic, and Roman medicine, beginning in the fifth century BCE and extending to the third century CE.* This era opens with the Greek physician Hippocrates of Cos (–460 to –370), and closes with the Roman physician Galen (+129– +199/216). This absurdly long piece of history is held together by the persistent attempt on the part of numerous authors to make medicine literate, that is, to record, analyze, and theorize about the work of healing in written books. The work of healing wounds and treating disease first appears in the Hellenic world, as it does in most early societies, as folk practice and as religious ritual. Specialists in this work appear in the *Iliad*: The "peerless physician," Machaon, son of Asklepios, demigod of healing, is summoned from the ranks of noble warriors to treat the arrow wound of King Menelaus. He draws the arrow, sucks out the blood, and applies "soothing remedies" (*epia pharmaka*).[1] Later in the epic, Patroclus, a layman, does an equally creditable job of arrow removal.[2] In the *Odyssey*, Odysseus' bleeding wound is staunched not by medication but by incantation, a religious healing ritual.[3] These two forms of healing persist together throughout the classical period. The healers who use soothing remedies evolve into the physicians of the classical era; the cantors remain practitioners of magical and religious healing. Healing work was caught up in the flowering of eloquence and inquiry that began on the Ionian coast in the fifth century BCE and began to evolve into "rational medicine," based on empirical observation and logical reasoning. Healing began to be called an *art* or *skill* (*techne*) and its practitioners *craftsmen* (*demiourgoi*),

---

*When clarity is required about dates. I shall use the convention of a minus sign (–) to designate centuries before the common era (BCE) and a plus sign (+) for centuries after the beginning of the common era (CE).

1

but it was equally a form of learning (*paideia*). Within the next few centuries, this new medicine spread around the Mediterranean basin.[4]

The new medicine takes literate shape in a collection of some 70 treatises known as the Hippocratic Collection. At the end of the millennium, Alexandrine scholars attributed the collection to Hippocrates of the Asklepiads, scion of a family of healers claiming the demigod Asklepios as their ancestor, and to his school of medicine on the island of Cos. The collection is a medley of works with little in common but the Ionic dialect in which they are written and the intent to explain the nature and course of disease, and the means of healing. In this collection, which was probably written over some five centuries, several treatises are devoted to the ways in which physicians should behave as they apply their medical skills: *Precepts*, *Art*, *Law*, *Decorum*, *Physician*, and, most renowned, *Oath*.[5]

What may be the earliest statement about ethics appears not in these ethical treatises but in a thoroughly clinical and epidemiological book titled *Epidemics I*, a book that is attributed by some modern scholars to Hippocrates himself.[6] *Epidemics I* presents a series of clinical cases, together with a description of the climate and geography of the places where the cases occurred. In the midst of this clinical reportage, the earliest admonition about the ethics of the practitioner appears in enigmatic form. The author is discussing the prognostic importance of the clinical sign of "coction of the evacuations" (thick, irritating discharges from the eyes, nose, bladder, bowels, and lungs). He states that coctions signify the nearness of crisis, the turn from disease toward health, and that the absence of coction portends pain, prolonged illness, and death. Then come the words, seemingly out of context, "Declare the past, diagnose the present, foretell the future. As to diseases, make a habit of two things—to help and not to harm. The art has three factors, the disease, the patient, the physician. The physician is the servant of the art. The patient must co-operate with the physician in combating the disease." The text immediately returns to its clinical tone with a discussion of pain and fever.[7]

The central maxim of this passage, "to help and not to harm," despite its enigmatic setting, seems clear, even banal. Galen, the greatest interpreter of Hippocrates, found the maxim almost insulting in its simplicity: why should it be necessary to command physicians not to harm their patients? He changed his mind, he says, only after seeing the incompetent work of many of his colleagues.[8] The medical historian Ludwig Edelstein saw these curt words as a sober command for a good physician to achieve the objective of his art.[9] Another historian suggests that it reflects the vivid awareness of healers that their therapeutic efforts—bleeding, cutting, burning, and the use of drugs—were dangerous and feared by the public and that such an imperative represented a public invitation to trust.[10] When quoted in modern contexts, it serves as a reminder that physicians should assess the possibilities of harm that attend any attempt to heal.[11]

None of these interpretations quite suit the original context. *Epidemics I* is a book about prognosis; barely a word is said about treatment. The clinical course of 42 patients is described; 25 of these cases end in death. The author's purpose is to teach physicians to recognize the sequence of symptoms in certain environments so that "these may be duly weighed when considering and deciding who is suffering from one of these diseases in an acute, fatal form or whether the patient may recover."[12] The essential function of the learned practitioner is to "declare the future" in relation to past and present signs. Prognosis is the heart of the Hippocratic art.

Another text, *Prognostic*, extolls the excellence of skilled prognosis. This exhaustive treatise on symptomatology opens with a short preface in which the "good physician" is described as one who can distinguish between a disease that is fatal and a disease from which the patient will recover, for in this way patients will respect him and entrust themselves to him for treatment. "You will be blameless if you learn and declare beforehand those who will die and those who will get better."[13] In the context of prognostication, helping and not harming means that the physician should undertake care only when "the disease does not exceed the strength of men's bodies" and the patient can benefit from medical ministrations.[14]

The same notion appears in *Art*, a book apparently written by a layman rather than a practitioner. The author states his conception of medicine in trenchant phrases; "it removes the suffering of the sick, lessens the violence of their diseases and does not attempt to cure those who are mastered by their diseases, realizing that in such cases medicine is powerless."[15] In defending medicine as a true art, the author exclaims, "If one demands from an art a power over what does not pertain to that art, or from nature a power over what does not belong to nature, his error is more like insanity than ignorance . . . so, if a man suffers from an ill too strong for the means at the disposal of medicine, he must not expect that it will be mastered by medicine." The author concludes that the experienced physician should never be blamed for refusing to take on desperate cases.[16] In this light, the "harm" mentioned in *Epidemics I* consists in subjecting to the rigors of medicine those who have no chance to recover. Finding those patients whose disease is susceptible to the physician's skill—patients who are able "to cooperate with the physician in combating the disease"—is the essence of the art and its ethic. In so doing, the physician benefits and does no harm. "To help and do no harm" are infinitives, which in Greek can stand for imperatives. The tone of the maxim is clearly deontological: it issues an order. In the context of prognostication, it implies that patients would be wronged by a physician who either predicted incorrectly or who, knowing the correct prognosis, undertook to do what he knew he could not accomplish. One modern commentator notes, "Hippocrates was showing the physician at the same time how to treat the patient and how to behave morally."[17]

Oath is most commonly cited as the compendium of the physician's ethic. Its origin is unknown. Once thought to have come from the hand of Hippocrates himself for use as an initiation rite into the clan of "the sons of Asklepios," this story of *Oath*'s origin is not supported by modern scholarship. Fifty years ago, Ludwig Edelstein suggested an interpretation that both clarified the origin and meaning of *Oath* and, at the same time, deepened the scholarly controversy. Edelstein proposed that *Oath* did not represent any widespread covention among physicians in the Greek world but was the private covenant of a small group of physicians who were followers of the philosopher, mystic, and mathematician Pythagoras. Edelstein contended that each phrase of the document could be related to dogmas of the Pythagorean faith that forbade the shedding of blood, the killing of the fetus, and the taking of life. This interpretation explains the odd fact that, while *Oath* forbids physicians to cause death or perform abortions, physicians in the classical world seem to have done both with impunity.[18] Only the Pythagorean faithful, Edelstein argued, would have refrained.

In this interpretation, *Oath* stems not from the exigencies of medical work or from the need to promote the physician's reputation, but from a genuine and articulate system of moral belief.[19] This religiously grounded moral seriousness contrasts, in Edelstein's view, with the rest of the so-called ethical content of the Hippocratic literature. The physician who appears in that literature is simply a prudent craftsman concerned with building a reputation as a trustworthy and skilled healer. All ethical advice aims to enhance his reputation and thus his business.[20] Despite its explanatory appeal, many contemporary scholars judge Edelstein's interpretation of *Oath* and of the ethics of Greek physicians as too "simplistic a model" to use in understanding the complex cultural and literary world of ancient medicine. They claim that it draws too much from the murky remains of Pythagoreanism and neglects equally plausible interpretations of its phrases based on popular morality.[21]

Whatever its origin, *Oath* is a striking example of deontology.[22] Oaths, vows, and promises are quintessential deontological acts: they bind the person to his word, as testified before a higher being. The Greek word for oath, *orkos*, is derived from a linguistic root meaning, "constraint." Oaths were prominent in Greek law, popular religion, and personal life. Oaths were taken solemnly and observed stringently. A deity in the Greek pantheon named Orkos, son of Eris ("wrath"), punished perjurers. The Hippocratic document is a typical oath: it begins by calling the divinities of health as witnesses, makes a promise of fidelity to one's teachers, lists six behaviors that the oath taker binds himself to avoid, and ends with an acceptance of the rewards and punishments entailed by observance or violation of the precepts. The first injunction is almost identical to the maxim of *Epidemics I*: "I will use treatment to help the sick according to my ability and judgment and never to bring them harm or injustice." This phrase is followed with the affirmation "I will never give a poison to anyone to cause death, not even if asked." These words, which are today often understood as a prohibition of euthanasia, could equally refer to the misuse of medical skills by physicians as accomplices in murder.[23] Physicians are slandered as "unpunished killers" not only in ancient comedy but also in serious historical and legal writings, and the notion must not have been far from the popular mind. One historian writes, "we may well understand why some physicians . . . felt urged to secure their professional and personal situation by swearing an Oath that could actually help, for instance, in a trial concerning death by poison." In a judicial speech prosecuting a physician as a poison murderer, the prosecutor exclaimed, "physicians who stand to the oaths sworn by themselves are bound to help and not to harm."[24]

Oath then repeats, in different words, the early injunction against harm that had echoed the maxim of *Epidemics I*: "into whatever houses I enter, I will enter to help the sick, and I will abstain from all intentional injustice and harm, especially from abusing the bodies of man or woman, bond or free." The injunction to refrain from "harm or intentional injustice" to one's patients, repeated three times in the ethical texts, is a central deontological element of Greek medical ethics. The two repetitions in *Oath* go further than the terse maxim of *Epidemics I*: they envision a medicine that, in addition to prognosis, has powerful and dangerous means of treatment. The physician is, in the words of the Homeric epics, the "healer with soothing remedies." The adjective *soothing* that often qualifies the word *pharmakon* reflects the ambiguity of that word, which can mean, in Greek, "therapeutic drug," "poison," or "charm."[25] Even though much of the classical pharmacopeia was mild and certain schools of classical physicians avoided drug therapies in favor of diet and exercise, some powerful drugs were in use, and the therapies of surgery, cautery, and bleeding were inherently dangerous and called for great prudence in their application. Indeed, in light of the prevailing theories of disease, almost any therapy could be dangerous, since the delicate balance of humors could be disrupted by any intervention if improperly chosen.[26] Two Hippocratic treatises on orthopedics, *Fractures* and *Joints*, reveal the influence of the maxim on primitive surgery. The author, who shows particular concern about mitigating pain during operations, comments on the frequent use by charlatans and even by decent practitioners of procedures that will do more harm than good.[27] The authors of the Hippocratic literature are acutely aware that the work (*techne*) of the Greek physician was inherently dangerous.

This central imperative has a poetic and a philosophical echo that takes it even deeper into Greek moral life. An ancient legend, related by the poet Pindar and repeated by Plato in the *Republic*, tells that Zeus, king of the gods, cast a lethal thunderbolt at the demigod patron of medicine, Asklepios, who, lured by a promise of monetary reward, undertook to heal a man whom the gods had marked for death. The moral of Pindar's poem is "From the gods we must expect things that suit our mortal minds, aware of the here and now, aware of our allotment: do not yearn, O my soul, for immortal life."[28] Plato rejects Pindar's version of the tale, claiming that, if Asklepios was the son of a god, he could not have been avaricious. Plato wishes to draw another lesson from the legend of Asklepios: true "sons of Asklepios" would never treat someone whom they knew was incurable, "though he were rich as Midas." Rather, they would minister to those who were basically healthy and suffering from a specific curable ailment; bodies diseased through and through, they would leave to die. This, says Plato, "is best for the patients and for the state." Asklepios and those who follow his practice can be called "statesmen."[29] The word translated as "statesman" is *politicos*, a person committed to the welfare of the *polis*, the Greek city-state. The *iatros politicos*, or statesman-physician, looks to the good of the community as he makes decisions about treatment. This Platonic passage suggests our use of the phrase *politic ethics*. The idea of an ethic that considers the relation between medicine and the society will grow in importance over the centuries, and the meaning of politic ethics will evolve in strange ways.

This Platonic idea reflects the Hippocratic rule about refraining from treating those whose recovery is unlikely. This rule may appear to be nothing more than prudence, for one's reputation as a healer depends more on one's successes than one's failures. Indeed, this motive appears again and again in traditional medical ethics, and led Ludwig Edelstein to judge that the professional ethics of the Greek physician "consist in doing his task well, in perfecting his skill; it is an ethic of outward achievement rather than of inner intention."[30] However, the rule goes beyond prudence to a profound ethical dimension of Greek life: the moral danger of overstepping human limits set by the gods or by nature. *Hybris*, overweening pride, is the primary human vice, and those in constant touch with life and death should be particularly careful to cultivate its opposite: *sophrosyne*, wise moderation. Asklepios, son of Apollo, had committed the sin of *hybris* and was punished by Zeus: he was not *sophron*, wisely moderate, in his zeal to heal and his desire for profit. Thus, the central imperative of *Oath* can be read at three levels of meaning: as a maxim of prudence, as a recognition of the limits of the art of medicine, and as a reflection of one of the fundamental moral beliefs of Greek culture.

Asklepios of Pindar's poem was not *sophron*. *Sophrosyne* is a virtue, fostering self-control and spurning self-indulgence. Aristotle describes the *sophron* as a person who "desires moderately the things that are pleasant." He praises this moderation as the virtue that "safeguards practical reason," which is the highest moral virtue whereby "one understands what is good for oneself and for men in general."[31] The Hippocratic literature recommends that the physician cultivate *sophrosyne* in daily intercourse with patients. The short essay entitled *Physician* advises the physician to look healthy and to be clean and well dressed so that he will be pleasing to patients. Then the author asserts, "as a prudent man [*sophron*], he should be of regular life and discreet in speech, grave and kind to all, in effect, a gentleman." The word *gentleman*, in Greek *kalokagathos*, is composed of the two Greek words for *beautiful* and *good*, and the phrase "beautiful and good" was commonly used to commend an individual as moral and upright.[32] The chapter urges the physician to have "a serious but not harsh countenance, for harshness is taken for arrogance and unkindness, while a man of uncontrolled laughter and excessive gaiety is considered vulgar . . . he must be just toward all." The author then notes that the sick put themselves "into the hands of their physicians in an intimate way and, in so doing, physicians encounter wives and maidens and precious possessions, "toward which self-control [*sophrosyne*] must be exercised."[33] This passage recalls the injunction of *Oath* never to do "intentional injustice in any house I may enter," particularly by sexual exploitation of its inhabitants. Again, by virtue of his work, the physician can endanger not only his patients' bodies but also their persons.

The book entitled *Decorum* opens with praise of wisdom: "The physician must be a lover of wisdom, that is, a philosopher, and so will be godlike."[34] The godlike wisdom, however, is quickly applied to mundane manners: the good practitioner will, by appearance, speech, and comportment, put the patient at ease and engender confidence. The way in which the physician determines his fee and speaks about it to the patient is related to the effects on the patient's health and confidence: "if you begin by discussing fees, you will suggest to the patient that you will go away . . . if no agreement is reached, or that you will neglect him and not prescribe any immediate treatment. So one must not be anxious about fixing a fee."[35] Also, the physician should consider the financial status of the patient: "sometimes give your services for nothing . . . if there be an opportunity of serving a stranger in financial straits, give full assistance."[36] The text then turns philosophical again, with a maxim that will have a long history in medical ethics, "for where there is love of mankind [*philanthropia*], there is love of the art [*philotechnia*]." Sir William Osler found in that phrase the very essence of medical ethics.[37] Yet the passage of time and the vagaries of translation may have inflated its meaning. The word *philanthropia*, translated grandly as "love of humankind," did come into philosophical prominence in Stoic philosophy and may carry its deeper moral weight in the works of a later writer on medical ethics, Scribonius Largus, but in *Decorum* it may mean something rather pedestrian, such as "if people like you and you like them, you will love your work and so will they."[38] The other ethical treatises of the Hippocratic collection, *Precepts*, *Law*, and *Art*, follow *Physician* and *Decorum* in describing the demeanor that the physician should maintain in dealing with patients. The bedside manner described in these treatises has remained almost unchanged throughout the centuries.

The decorum of the physician will enhance his reputation (*doxa*). The English word *reputation* does not quite catch the subtlety of *doxa*, which designates not the self-advertising that we associate with the word *reputation* but rather the reflection of the inner self to others, the external manifestation of moral virtue. The anonymous authors of the Hippocratic texts were aware of the moral ambiguity which lurks behind the praise of public conduct. Their words can be read as commending a set of practiced behaviors, a style and a manner, that will win and preserve a good reputation, "Such being the things that make for good reputation," says *Decorum*.[39] This will bring patients to them. But there is a more properly

moral motive, which the authors note as well. The physician's behavior and reputation are also beneficial to the patient: "some patients, though conscious that their
condition is perilous, recover their health simply through their contentment with
the goodness of the physician."[40] The authors of these texts also know that reputation can be fallacious. "Many are physicians by repute," says *Law*, "but few are
physicians in reality." The physician in reality is one who has natural ability and
has devoted himself to serious study of the art, and, indeed, the one who truly
understands the art must be "holy," for "holy things, i.e., the knowledge of medicine, are revealed only to holy men."[41] *Oath* solemnly declares, "I keep pure and
holy my life and my art."[42]

The decorum literature has occasional dashes of philosophy. Some scholars
find hints of the sophist Protagoras in *Art*.[43] *Law* may have been written by someone under Stoic influence, although "the internal evidence is very slight."[44] There
is something of a Stoic flavor to *Decorum*, although some scholars see a tinge of
Epicureanism, and Edelstein recognizes a medical version of Aristotelian virtue
ethics.[45] *Physician*, short as it is, is redolent of popular morality, and the difficult
and obscure *Precepts*, while containing a word, *philanthropia*, that carries great
weight in the ethical vocabulary of Stoicism, hardly rises above popular morality
and prudent advice. Thus, in a world where ethical philosophies flourished, the
medical ethical literature does not reflect many of the ideas and arguments of those
philosophies other than what might be expected from cultured writers. Indeed,
Plato, Aristotle, the Stoics, and the Epicureans seem more impressed by Hippocrates than Hippocrates and his colleagues are by the philosophers.[46]

The Hippocratic ethic, then, consists of two powerful deontological pieces, the
maxim of *Epidemics I* and *Oath*, and an ample exposition of decorum that can be
seen either as mere etiquette or as an ethic of virtue and character. There is almost
nothing in the Hippocratic literature that fits what we called, in our introduction,
politic ethics. Although we derived the term *politic ethics* from Plato's praise of
Asklepios as a statesman who looked to the good of the state to guide the healing
art, almost no politic ethics of medicine appears in the classical world.

A politic ethics would explicate the physician's social responsibility to patients
as a class, to colleagues, and to society and the state. Yet the extant literature has
only rare references to these responsibilities. The Hippocratic texts do not mention any duty to serve all persons in need of medical attention. Plato suggests that
citizen physicians treated citizens, while their assistants cared for slaves, but otherwise there is little evidence to support this picture of a barrier between classes.
One commentator goes so far as to say, "In none of the many treatises of the Hippocratic Collection is the least distinction made between slaves and free men."[47] The
duty to treat the victims of epidemics is not mentioned in the medical literature,
but it is suggested by the historian Thucydides in his history of the plague at Athens in –430.[48] No obligation to care for enemies can be found. Indeed, Hippocrates
is said to have explicitly refused to treat Persians.[49] Relationships between physi-

cians are discussed only in terms of the duty to one's teachers,[50] the propriety of consultation in difficult cases, and the impropriety of jealously.[51] Quacks, who are ignorant of the art, are disdained.[52] Although "Sons of Asklepios" is a common appellation for physicians, there does not appear to have been anything like a profession.[53] Possibly some clubs or fraternities of practitioners existed. If Edelstein's interpretation of *Oath* is credited, a sodality of Pythagorean physicians may have existed in Graeca Magna. The ancient world knew no regulation or licensure for physicians. *Law* opens with the remark that "medicine is the only art which our states have made subject to no penalty save that of dishonor," suggesting that the civil laws imposed little obligation on practitioners. Both Aristotle and Plato briefly comment on how physicians should be treated by the courts, suggesting that their skills and knowledge require special consideration: Plato suggests that a physician who deliberately intends to do harm by poisoning should be put to death; Aristotle suggests that the medical failures of physicians should be judged not by any citizen juror but only by persons educated in medicine.[54] The relationship between the state and physicians is only vaguely suggested.

The story thus far has lingered in the Greek world; it must go further. Legend tells that the demigod Asklepios arrived in Rome to repel the plague of −295. In fact, his human namesake, an Alexandrine Greek named Asclepiades, brought literate medicine to Rome around −120. He found in sober Rome a folk medicine of myths and simples, administered by the *paterfamilias* rather than by physicians. The theories of Greek medicine and its fancy practitioners were derided by such sturdy Romans as Pliny Elder and Cato. Asclepiades "was influenced by his Roman environment and was Roman in practical application of medicine."[55] A prolific writer, he helped "mature our beneficial profession," as one of his most prominent successors, Celsus, wrote.[56] The "beneficial profession" (*salutaris professio* can also mean "healing profession") flourished largely among the nobility and the wealthy classes. Few Romans appear to have been attracted to medical practice. The majority of physicians in Roman lands were foreigners, many of them former slaves of Greek origin.[57]

Latin literature about medicine was predominantly practical rather than theoretical. Two of the most prominent Latin books of medicine were written by laymen, Celsus and Pliny Elder.[58] Another practical book, a pharmacological text entitled *Compositiones*, was written by Scribonius Largus (c. +14–54), probably a Greek freedman and, for part of his career, a military physician with the armies of the Emperor Claudius in Britain. This book opens with a remarkable contribution to the ethics of medicine. Scribonius, arguing in favor of the therapeutic use of drugs, comments that physicians who administer drugs must have certain moral qualities.

> All gods and men should hate the physician whose heart lacks compassion and the
> spirit of human kindness [*humanitas*]. These very qualities preclude the physician,
> bound by the sacred oath [*sacramentum*] of medicine, from giving a harmful drug

even to an enemy—yet the physician will attack that same enemy, when occasion demands, in his role as a soldier and good citizen.

Scribonius then refers to *Oath*, which "prepared his [Hippocrates'] students' hearts and minds to learn humane feelings." He notes that Hippocrates prohibited physicians from performing abortions because "how much more evil would he, who thought it wrong to destroy even the tenuous possibility of a man, judge the harming of a living human being." Scribonius, recalling the maxim of *Epidemics I*, says, "medicine is the science of healing, not of harming."[59]

This passage is remarkable for several reasons. First, it explicitly alludes to *Oath*, which is rarely cited in the classical medical literature. Second, it equates the medical oath with the *sacramentum* of the Roman soldier, the military oath to defend emperor and empire with one's life. Third, it is reminiscent of the ethics of late Stoicism. *Humanitas*, the Latin equivalent of the Greek *philanthropia*, was a primary virtue of Stoic philosophy: the recognition that all humans, of every nature and condition, were equal in one universal commonwealth. The physician's service to the sick must transcend human enmity.[60] Scribonius' striking invocation of the Hippocratic ethic seems to have had little subsequent influence. Although Scribonius' pharmacopoeia was frequently copied throughout the ages, the moral exhortation of the preface seems to have gone unnoticed until recently.

The premier figure in preserving and amending the Hippocratic tradition was Galen (+129–200), a native of Pergamum who practiced in Rome. Among his voluminous writings are many treatises and commentaries on ethics. In a short essay, "The Best Doctor Is Also a Philosopher," Galen asserts that any doctor worthy of the name made honorable by Hippocrates must "know all parts of philosophy: the logical, the physical and the ethical." He must be skilled at reasoning about the problems presented to him, must understand the nature and function of the body within the physical world, and must "practice temperance and despise money: all evil actions that men undertake are done either at the prompting of greed or under the spell of pleasure." Galen's philosophical doctor is not merely a student of philosophical literature but one whose life has been formed by justice, and temperance. He will possess all other virtues since, according to Stoic doctrine, "all the virtues are connected as if by one string." At many points in his voluminous writings, Galen excoriates physicians for avarice, contentiousness, and ignorance. The ideal physician treats the poor and follows a medical regimen dictated by rationality. He is a student of all that affects health. He is fair-minded, and lives a modest, even ascetic life. Galen cites the Hippocratic decorum literature to justify this picture of the good physician. It is obvious here, and in other writings, that Galen sees himself in this picture (although he was accused of fleeing plague-ridden Rome and was reputed to have been an irascible and proud man). He reports that many physicians were hostile to him "because of his medical skills and his dignified way of life."[61]

Galen is silent on *Oath* unless one accepts as genuine an Arabic commentary on *Oath* sometimes attributed to him. That commentary stresses the physician's behavior in the presence of the sick and does not emphasize the more deontological injunctions of *Oath* on suicide, abortion, and euthanasia. The etiquette of the physician in dealing with the patient is explained under the headings "entrance, words, appearances, dress, hair, nails, smell." The Galenic etiquette has a moral purpose, says one historian: "to convince the patient that the Hippocratic healer who stands before him or her is the person who can cure," for "in the battle against illness the patient's cooperation is essential for success."[62] Galen also wrote a handbook for persons choosing a physician, "On Examining the Best Physician." One should look for a learned physician, a perennial student, and a man of very regular life. The ethics of the Galenic physician focus primarily on the character of those who would practice medicine. Learning and study are primary, regularity of life is essential, and politeness and graciousness toward patients is a powerful instrument of healing. Galen teaches a decorum ethic, stressing attitudes and virtues rather than rules and duties. His picture of the ethical physician endures down the ages, incorporated constantly in the medieval and Renaissance treatises on the good physician.

We know little about the actual behavior of physicians in classical times. A few were infamous: a court physician, C. Stertinius Xenophon, was implicated in the murder of the Emperor Claudius by his wife, Agrippina. Many were maligned. The old Roman chauvinist, Cato, claimed that all Greek physicians were out to murder with medicine all non-Greeks. Constant barbs about physicians being unpunished killers appear in comedy and satire. The greed of physicians is upbraided. Pliny Elder says, "the worst thing a person can do is mention his physician in his will." Most famously, physicians appear in an unflattering light in Martial's *Epigrams*: "I was sick, but you, Dr. Symmachus, attended me with a train of 100 apprentices—one hundred hands, frosted by the north wind, have pawed me. I had no fever before, Symmachus, but I now have one."[63] Galen frequently excoriates many of his colleagues as ignorant, avaricious, and crude.

Over the centuries of classical medicine, the dominant themes of medical morality fall into the realm of moral discourse that we have called decorum. In the moral climate of the Hellenic-Hellenistic-Roman world, decorum, while it has much in common with what we today call etiquette, also touches the deeper moral qualities that we would also call virtues. The English word *decorum* is open to two quite different interpretations. Defined as "seemliness, propriety, etiquette; particular usage required by politeness or decency,"[64] decorum refers both to the more superficial conventions of politeness and to a deeper moral characteristic, decency. Obviously, a person can act decorously, putting on manners that will please, and yet be a scoundrel, prompting many moralists to ruminate on how external behavior is related to internal virtue. Cicero defines *decorum* as behavior that "ornaments" life, and he concludes that it is "manifested only when there is pre-existing moral rectitude (*cum antegressa est honestas*)."[65] This discussion will persist during the history of moral philosophy and, throughout the long tradition of medical ethics, the double connotation of the word will appear again and again: the external characteristics that render a physician acceptable to patients and enhance his reputation must be matched by an inner integrity and virtue. The picture of the decorous physician, from the earliest Hippocratic texts through Galen and even down to modern times, is remarkably constant. We have no way of knowing how often that literary picture was matched by reality. We may only wonder how many practitioners of healing did "keep pure and holy their life and art" by demonstrating the Hippocratic decorum in behavior and in belief.[66]

The deontological tone of the classical texts is much more muted than is the decorum. *Oath* is certainly a dictate of stringent duties, and its interpretation as a Roman military *sacramentum* by Scribonius makes it even more so. But, as we have seen, *Oath* is rarely noticed in the classical literature. It apparently did not have wide currency, and does not seem to have been actually sworn in any public ceremony, except perhaps by small coteries of like-minded physicians. Finally, the civic ethics of medicine emerges in minor ways. Legal sanctions for medical malpractice appear in Roman law.[67] Clubs or fraternities of like-minded physicians seem to have been popular, but almost nothing is known about them (they may have been secret societies). In Hellenistic and Roman times, cities appear to have appointed official civic physicians, but their role is unclear.[68] Cities often gave physicians exemptions from certain taxes and onerous civil duties, but the rationale for this civic recognition is poorly understood and mention of it appears in the legal rather than the medical literature.[69] The politic ethics of medicine, although somewhat more visible than in Hellenic times, is still undeveloped.

2

Medieval Medicine
Fifth to Fourteenth Centuries CE

The second great sweep of medical history begins at the end of the fourth century, with the founding of the first Christian hospital at Caesarea in Cappadocia, and concludes at the end of the fourteenth century, with medicine well ensconced in the universities and in the public life of the emerging nations of Europe. After Galen's magisterial summation and revision of Hippocratic medicine, literate medicine went stale for some five centuries, suffering the same fate as literature, the arts, and government in the general decay of the Western Roman Empire.[1] While medical scholarship continued to flourish in Alexandria and Constantinople, in the West literate medicine was confined to encyclopedias and formulaic collections.[2] Although the sources allow us elusive glimpses of secular physicians during the early Middle Ages, the practice of medicine increasingly became the purview of monks and other clergy, and only tattered remnants of classical literate medicine were preserved in monastic libraries.

During these centuries, the Christian faith, propagated by the Roman Catholic Church, permeated all aspects of life in the West. The very conception of medicine, as well as its practice, was deeply touched by the doctrine and discipline of the Church. This theological and ecclesiastical influence manifestly shaped the ethics of medicine, but it even indirectly affected its science since, as its missionaries evangelized the peoples of Western and Northern Europe, the Church found itself in a constant battle against the use of magic and superstition in the work of healing. It championed rational medicine, along with prayer, to counter superstition.

The Church looked favorably on medical healing because its teachings rested on the gospel of Jesus, called the Christ, who was himself described as a miraculous healer of the sick and who commanded his followers to attend the sick. Jesus said "Come . . . inherit the kingdom . . . for I was sick and you visited me," assimilating an act of mercy to a needy stranger to an act done to himself. These words became a command to his followers (Mt. 9; Mt. 10.8; Mt. 25:34–36). Jesus compares himself to a physician: asked why he consorted with sinners, he answers, "Those who are whole need not a physician, but those who are sick" (Mt. 9:12). Even though miracle and prayer were the instruments of healing in these Gospel texts, and physical healing was a metaphor for the healing of the soul by divine grace, human medicine benefited by the comparison. Early Christian believers, while acknowledging the providence of God in allowing sickness and affirming that healing came through God's beneficence, did not repudiate human healing. An occasional author, such as the somewhat heterodox Origen, denigrated human medicine in favor of divine healing, but the corpus of early Christian literature contains no repudiation of human medical wisdom and skill, or of medical remedies, both of which come from the divine power. Among the many affirmations in the writings of early Christian Fathers about the legitimacy of seeking medical help, the words of St. Basil of Cappadocia stand out: "we must take great care to employ the medical art, if it should be necessary, not as making it wholly accountable for our state of health or illness but as redounding to the glory of God . . . we should neither repudiate this art altogether nor does it behoove us to repose all our confidence in it . . . when reason allows, we call in the doctor but we do not leave off hoping in God."[3]

The early Church not only endorsed the use of human medicine, it also encouraged care of the sick as a work of charity. As early as the second century, comparison between the saving work of Jesus and the healing work of physicians had became common in Christian rhetoric: the designation *Christus Medicus* became familiar.[4] Many teachers recalled the parable told by Jesus of a stranger who, on encountering a wounded man, "had compassion upon him," provided medical care, and paid for his recovery (Luke 10:29–37).[5] St. John Chrysostom, writing in the fourth century, recalls that parable and tells his congregation, "It matters not whether the sick one is Christian, Jew or Gentile, rich or poor, slave or free: it is his need that calls out to you."[6] During the third century, when plague swept through Italy and North Africa, Christians became famous for their devotion to the stricken, even being nicknamed *Parabolani*, the reckless ones, for their willingness to risk their lives. In +251, Cyprian, bishop of Carthage wrote, "the pestilence searches out the justice of each and every one . . . whether the well care for the sick, whether relatives dutifully love their kinsmen as they should, whether masters show compassion for their ailing slaves, whether physicians do not desert the afflicted." Dionysius, bishop of Alexandria, attested that Christian people "showed unbounded love and loyalty, never sparing themselves and thinking only of others. Heedless of danger, they took charge of the sick, attending to their every need and ministering to them in Christ. . . . Many in nursing and curing others transferred their death to themselves and died in their stead." The pagans, he said, "at first onset of the disease pushed the sufferers away and fled from their dearest." It was, said Cyprian, the duty of Christians not only to cherish their own but to practice merciful kindness even to strangers and enemies. Emperor Julian the

Apostate, although disdainful of the Christian faith, had grudgingly acknowledged this expansive Christian charity: "These impious Galileans support not only their own poor but ours as well." One scholar suggests that the dedication of Christians during these devastating years contributed significantly to the extraordinary growth of the Christian Church during the third century: even the simplest nursing care certainly contributed to the survival of some victims more effectively than did abandonment. Christian belief provides a rationale for suffering and for charity that the prevailing pagan cults lacked, and many pagans, on seeing and receiving this Christian charity, were impressed to the point of conversion.[7]

In +372, St. Basil put his words about the utility of medicine into practice. As bishop of Caesarea in Cappadocia, he opened a hospital for lepers, served by nurses and medical attendants. His friend, St. Gregory of Nazianzus, wrote of this *xeno-dochion* (house for strangers), "This is a new city where disease is regarded in a religous light and sympathy put to the test . . . a treasure house of godliness. We no longer look on the fearful and pitiable sight of men like corpses before death . . . driven from cities, from public places, from water courses . . . Basil it was who took the lead in persuading men not to scorn their fellowmen, nor to dishonor Christ by their inhumanity toward human beings."[8] This hospital became a model for many similar institutions throughout the Christian world, where the work of caring for the sick was defined as a work of Christian compassion and service of God.[9] Monastic rules from the sixth century on commanded special solicitude for the sick—monks and laypersons alike. Places of hospitality, or hospices, were established in monastic communities everywhere. The father of Western monasticism, Cassiodorus, provided instructions for the care of the sick, including a bibliography of classical medical texts that the monastic physicians and infirmarians should study.[10]

The pious work of caring for the sick demanded some rudimentary skills of nursing and healing. Monastic infirmarians, often unlearned in literate medicine, became competent herbalists. Pharmacopeias were compiled. One of the most elaborate of these was *Liber Simplicis Medicinae* by the mystic and musical composer Hildegard, abbess of the convent of Bingen (1098–1179).[11] Handbooks prepared for the education of parish priests often included advice about medical assistance, along with instructions about ritual and pastoral duties. Medicine appears to have been cultivated in a more scholarly way in the cathedral schools of the eleventh century, precursors of the medieval universities. Bishop Fulbert (d. 1028), founder of the cathedral school of Chartres, appears to have been, among many other things, a competent medical scholar, ready to utilize the wisdom of Hippocrates while depending on the mercy of the Lord. "Earthly doctors," he wrote, "learn by long experience the power of herbs to alter the condition of the human body . . . yet no physician is so experienced as to escape absolutely incurable maladies, as Hippocrates, greatest of physicians testifies . . . Christ, author of heavenly medicine, could cure disease by mere command." The history of another medical bishop, Derold of Amiens, resembles a medical morality play: when he was poisoned by a jealous medical rival (a graduate of Salerno), he cured himself, poisoned his poisoner, and then deliberately cured him only partially, leaving him a cripple. Hardly edifying for a physician, much less a bishop.[12]

In the late eleventh century, a group of pious Italian merchants donated alms to support a hospital in Jerusalem for sick pilgrims to the Holy Land. Several of these donors took religious vows, calling themselves the Poor Brethren of the Hospital of St. John of Jerusalem, and devoted themselves to caring for the patients of their hospital. This tiny group "makes a vow which no other people make, promising to be the serf and slave of our lords, the sick." Their vow placed them as vassals under obedience to those whom they served. This reversal of the feudal hierarchy introduced into the work of healing the moral duty of service to the sick, a duty that had been only dimly affirmed in Hellenic medicine but that was clearly implied by Christian belief. Recognized by Pope Pascal II as a religious order in 1116, the Poor Brethren established hospitals along the pilgrimage route from Europe to the Holy Land. These hospitals followed a regimen not unlike that of the modern hospital: physicians were required to visit the beds of patients twice daily, a written record of the patient's progress and treatment was hung above the bed, pharmacies were established, concern for cleanliness and appropriate diet was sustained by rules, and, above all, the spiritual welfare of the sick was fostered. Care was provided to all in need, whether friend or foe. Ironically, this charitable order evolved into a mighty military order, renamed the Knights Hospitallers, whose brethren fought ferociously against the Saracens. They maintained their work for the sick, but the duties of war loomed large. One of their hospital administrators complained in 1296 that the Order's leaders were spending on armaments what "should have been spent for the benefit of our lords, the sick, to sustain them and the poor."[13]

The joining of military and medical activities may puzzle the modern mind, to which the brutality of military engagement seems quite incompatible with the compassion of medical care. Those vowed men who moved between shedding the blood of Saracens in battle to bloodletting in the hospital wards (even the fighting brethren were required to serve for at least a month in the hospital) apparently felt no conflict. Indeed, a book written for the edification of the Knights extols the virtue of courage and the virtue of hospitality as the two essential qualities required of the brethren of the Order: "Not only when pouring soothing ointment but when shedding blood, the brethren are at one and the same time valorous warriors and charitable hospitallers."[14] During the late Middle Ages, many other men and women (particularly women) formed religious congregations for the service of the sick and dying, serving the Hôtels Dieu that were established in many European towns.

The melding of medicine and Christian belief injected a strong deontological tone into the work of caring for the sick. The divine approbation of human heal-

ing, the model of Jesus as healer, his words equating a visit to the sick with a visit
to him, the linking of salvation to works of mercy for the needy, and the translation of these biblical notions into duties akin to obedience between lord and vas-
sal all introduced strong imperatives into the work of healing. Commands of the
Lord, obligations of vassals to their liege lords, the vows of monks and pious laypersons are all strongly deontological in nature. The deontological tone of the *Oath*
of Hippocrates fits into this culture of command and obligation but, in the early
Christian centuries, reference to it is rare. In the fourth century, St. Gregory of
Nazianzus' eulogy for his physician brother, Caesarius, remarked that he was so
beloved of his patients "that he did not need Hippocrates to administer an oath to
him."[15] Another Church Father, St. Jerome, advised a young priest to be chaste
of speech and eyes when he visited the sick, particularly women, recalling that
Hippocrates had given an oath for the guidance of his students, so "how much
more must we, charged with the cure of souls, love all Christians as our neigh-
bors."[16] The Hippocratic *Oath* appears somewhat more frequently in the medical
literature preserved in monastic texts from the eighth to the tenth centuries. While
rarely described in detail, *Oath* is recalled as imposing a rigorous duty: "he who
wishes to begin the art of medicine . . . ought to take the oath and not shrink in
any way from its consequences."[17] Some references to *Oath* stress the physician's
obligation to remain chaste in regard to women, and one widespread manuscript
refers to *Oath*'s prohibition of death-dealing medicines and abortion. A version
of *Oath*, amended "so that a Christian may take it," circulated before the tenth
century.[18] The Greek divinities are replaced by "God the Father of our Lord Jesus
Christ," the prohibition of abortion is strengthened, and the stricture against "cutting for the stone" is dropped. Although it is unknown how often or by whom the
classical or the Christian oath was taken, it represented a deontological document
congenial to Catholic physicians of the Middle Ages.[19]

The deontological tone of Catholic medicine was reinforced by the interest in
medicine taken by Church law. Canon law, made up of the decrees of Church
councils, bishops, and popes, becomes a dominant force in Church life after the
eleventh century. As early as 1139, Lateran Council II permitted monks to practice medicine within certain strict limitations. During the next century, many
Church councils and decrees addressed the practice of monastic medicine (a clerical
license to practice medicine was called *urere et secare*, "to burn and cut"). In 1215,
Lateran Council IV decreed that all Catholics must confess their sins to their parish priest, and in another canon it required physicians to admonish their patients
to summon "the physician of the soul" before they "apply bodily medicines."[20]
This intimate linking of spiritual with bodily medicine, under the command of
the Church, stimulated theologians and canonists to articulate the Christian duties of physicians.[21] Gradually, Church authorities restricted, almost to the point
of prohibition, the practice of medicine by clerics, opening more opportunities
for the growth of a lay profession. Clerical and lay physicians were held to high

moral standards. The extensive literature instructing priests how to deal with penitents lists the "sins of physicians": harming patients by ignorance or incompetence, advising treatment contrary to Church law or morals (e.g., by violating rules about fasting or by prescribing masturbation or extramarital coitus for presumed medical reasons), exploiting patients out of greed, and failing to warn of impending death. Abortion and contraception, prohibited by strict divine commands, could not be part of a physician's practice.[22] In this way, medicine and the work of physicians were surrounded by the deontology of divine law and ecclesiastical rules.

The deontology, however, did not overwhelm the decorum. The monastic medical manuscripts describe the role and character of the physician in terms almost identical to Hippocratic texts, such as *Decorum* and *Law*, adding ample citation of biblical texts. Physicians are admonished to be studious and of good moral character, cheerful and clean, gracious, reliable, and humble. "The greatest felicity," says one text, "is to keep things in balance, so that one is accomplished in the art and endowed with the best of manners."[23] Even in passages extolling the classical decorum, however, the Christian duty to serve the sick poor persistently appears: "The physician should not heal for the sake of gain, nor give more consideration to the rich than to the poor, or to the noble than to the ignoble."[24] The leading theologian of the thirteenth century, St. Thomas Aquinas, affirmed this obligation, although he recognized the difficulty of fulfilling it, since physicians who felt absolutely bound would be overwhelmed by poor patients and unable to make a living.[25] One of the leading surgeons of the next century, Henri de Mondeville, recommended prudent cost shifting: "Give advice to the poor for love of God only, but the wealthy should be made to pay dearly."[26]

In the sixth century, a militant faith called Islam appeared in Arabia, quickly spreading north into Syria and Persia and then west into Egypt. Originating in the inspired words of the prophet Mohammed (570–632), Islam not only taught a belief; it conquered lands and, assimilating the cultural and political forms of the Persian, Byzantine, and Egyptian lands that it occupied, achieved by the ninth century heights of splendor in the arts, literature, science, and medicine. Islam was a monotheistic faith with a complex moral teaching. The Koran prescribed a form of life for the faithful: forgiveness, moderation, honesty, humility, kindness, and brotherhood among believers, toleration of nonbelievers, and all this as a duty to Allah, the Beneficent and Compassionate. In addition to the Koran, the *hadith*, stories from the life of the prophet, provided exemplars of behavior. Around this ethical core, interpretations and particular rulings were incorporated into a body of law both judicial and moral, *Shari'a*, or "The Way toward Water." As Arab scholarship expanded and turned to science and medicine, this living religious ethics was bound to be felt.[27]

In the ninth century, the literate medicine of classical culture began to flow again into the West from Constantinople through the great Muslim cities of

Baghdad, Damascus, Cairo and the brilliant Islamic society of Andalusia in Spain. Credit for the preservation of classical medicine must be attributed to the center of scholarship at Jundi-Shapur in southern Persia. Founded by King Shapur I in +260, this small city attracted Christian and Zoroastrian scholars and, in +490, was enlarged by an influx of Persian Nestorian Christians who were given shelter after being expelled from Edessa by the Byzantine Emperor Zeno. The Nestorians brought a rich library of theological and medical books, including Syriac versions of the Hippocratic literature and the works of Galen. In 529 a scholarly immigration of Neo-Platonists, expelled from Athens as pagans, joined the faculty. Jewish scholars from Mesopotamia were welcomed to the ecumenical campus. Missions from Jundi-Shapur traveled to India to study Hindu medicine and philosophy.

After the Muslim conquest of Persia, the caliphs favored the scholarship of Jundi-Shapur until attention shifted to the great urban center of Baghdad. For six centuries, Greek, Jewish, Christian, Persian, Muslim, and Hindu ideas, both medical and religious, flourished at this extraordinary university. Its college of translators rendered the great works of antiquity into Persian and Arabic, and its hospital (*bimaristan*) trained physicians who served throughout the Near East. One early royal patron, King Nushirvan, convened a medical congress to discuss the best methods of treatment. The medical ethics of the Jundi-Shapur tradition are summarized in the words of one of its leading professors, a physician, philosopher, and politician, Burzuya: "I read in medical books that the best physician is one who gives himself over to his profession. . . . I exerted myself in the treatment of patients. Those whom I could not cure, I tried to make their sufferings more bearable. . . . From no one whom I treated did I demand any fee or reward."[28]

Practical Ethics of the Physician (Abad al-Tib), written by the ninth-century physician Ishaq ibn 'Ali al-Ruhawi, may be the first treatise devoted exclusively to medical ethics in the Islamic tradition. It clearly demonstrates a wealth of scholarship and a depth of ethical perception, as well as practical familiarity with medical practice. Twenty-one chapters present comprehensive principles and suggestions about the behavior of physicians, patients, family, visitors, and caretakers. Hippocrates, Galen, Aristotle, and a host of Greek and Islamic philosophers are often cited. The book opens with a treatise on God, the creator of nature and the granter of reason, whereby humans can understand the body and soul. The physician is then admonished that, since his body is the receptacle for the spirit, his first duty is to maintain his own health. The physician must also refresh his soul by prayer and by reading spiritual and scientific books. After a long dissertation on anatomy and physiology (which may have been interpolated by another author), al-Ruhawi describes the characteristics that a virtuous physician shows when dealing with patients: mercy, conscientious attention, patience, and firmness. He should be chaste, keep secrets, and bestow the benefits of his science "on all people without distinguishing them as to friend or foe, in agreement or disagreement." Physicians may earn an honest living by their work, but they must ensure that "they use justice to the poor and weak so that the benefits of the medical art be universal and similar for the strong and the weak." The most essential truth for a physician to remember is that "The philosopher can only improve the soul but the virtuous physician can improve both soul and body. The physician is imitating the acts of Allah, the Exalted, as much as he can." The author intersperses his admonitions and arguments with anecdotes, "some of which are amusing," to illustrate ethical practice. Al-Ruwahi also describes an elaborate examination to qualify physicians for practice that probed not only knowledge of the classics of medicine but also the moral understanding of the candidate. Such examinations were, as we know, applied in the administration of medical practice in the caliphates. Al-Ruwahi's *Practical Ethics* is a rich compendium of medical decorum and deontology, although it is more of a syncretistic work than a pure example of Islamic ethics.[29]

Three Islamic physicians were particularly influential in medical science, Rhazes, Ahwazi (Haly Abbas), and Ibn Sina (Avicenna). Each wrote ethical treatises that, in general, recall the Hippocratic decorum but emphasize strongly two ideas that are not in the Hippocratic tradition: the ultimate power of God over life, death, and healing and the obligation to care for the poor. Avicenna's highly influential *Canon of Medicine* opens with an eloquent treatise on the place of medicine within the human community. Medicine, says Avicenna, can be seen in three ways: as the pursuit of a practical art, rewarded by money; as the practice of devotion to one's needy fellow humans, rewarded by gratitude from those who have experienced the physician's generosity and, finally, as devotion to God, which has a dual reward: the good of the patient who is cured and the good of the physician who, touched by divine love, is granted insight into the realities of nature.[30] In addition to its scholarly literature, medieval Islamic culture developed a highly organized medical system. Charitable hospitals were associated with major mosques. Medical education, examination, and licensure of physicians were established as early as the tenth century in the caliphates.[31]

Jewish life in the Diaspora flourished in Mesopotamia and, when that land came under Islamic rule, Jewish scholarship continued to thrive. Jewish physicians were welcomed in the caliphates and participated in the scholarly renaissance of medicine in Islam. The Torah, revealed by Yahweh as the law for the people of Israel, contains a few texts referring to the healing work of physicians. Two of these texts seemed contradictory: Exodus 15:26 says, "I will put none of the diseases upon thee [Israel], for I am the Lord that healeth thee," while Exodus 21:27 states, "if men quarrel and one smites another with a stone and he die not but must keep to bed . . . he [the smiter] must cause him to be thoroughly healed." In the first text, Yahweh is the healer; in the second, some human agent is presumably given the task. The rabbinical commentators debated the apparent contradiction and reached the opinion that, even though Yahweh inflicts illness and takes it away, He also gives permission to humans to act as intermediaries. A text from the Book of

Wisdom of Ben Sira (also known as Ecclesiasticus) persuaded the rabbis that human medicine comes from the hand of God, "Honor the physician . . . from God the physician gets his wisdom. . . . God brings forth medicines from the earth and let a prudent man not ignore them" (Ecclus. 39:1).[32] The Mishna, the first great commentary on the Torah, contains an extensive discussion of the diagnosis of leprosy for the purpose of priestly declaration of ritual impurity. The Babylonian and Palestinian Talmuds and many other ancient commentaries on the Torah deal more extensively with illness, healing, birth, and death. In the Jewish cultural tradition, the role of physician was greatly honored. An oath, attributed to Asaph Judeus, who lived in Syria in the sixth century, places the physician's duties in the context of covenant and Torah. The physician must be "mindful of the Lord God of all flesh and seek Him in truth, uprightness, and rectitude." The physician must take care not to kill any man with the drugs he administers or give a drug that would cause an abortion for a woman pregnant by adultery. He must not covet wealth or any depraved sexual commerce. These and many other injunctions are "a commandment of the Torah and it behooves us to perform it with all our heart and soul." *Propaedeutic for Physicians*, by Isaac Israeli, a tenth-century opthalmologist of great fame, opens with the claim that since man is made in the image of God, he has the obligation "to make use of all things to ensure his being, his continuance, and his preservation." In 48 short maxims, the author sketches a physician who is learned, honest, cautious, and compassionate to the poor. The physician's prudence should range from the profound to the practical: "Medicine is concerned about the possible rather than the necessary. Death is certain and unavoidable: it is outside the power of the physician. . . . The physician should determine fees with the patient while sickness is serious. Otherwise, when he improves he will forget what you have done for him."[33]

One of the greatest Talmudists was also one of history's greatest physicians. Moses ben Maimon, or Maimonides (1135–1204), holds as high a place in the history of philosophy and religion as in the history of medicine. Born and educated in Cordova, he settled in Cairo, where he studied medicine and eventually became so renowned a physician that he was chosen as personal doctor by the Sultan Saladin. He vividly describes a day in his practice, beginning with hours of attendance on his royal patients. Then he returned home for lunch (which he could not take at the palace lest he violate Jewish dietary law), to find his waiting room filled with common people seeking his help, as well as Jewish scholars seeking his wisdom. A prolific author, Maimonides composed a major commentary on the Talmud, a philosophical work of enduring value, *Guide to the Perplexed*, and many medical works, including translations of the works of Galen, Hippocrates, and Avicenna. His writings as a Talmudic scholar occasionally touch ethical questions of great importance for medicine. He argues strongly that the saving of life justifies the suspension of religious laws, such as the observance of Sabbath; he supports a religious duty to assist those who are wounded, sick, or drowning; and he expounds on medically assisted abortion and on the determination of death. In his medical writings, he is concerned about the virtues of the physician. In his *Treatise on Asthma*, for example, he includes a lovely essay on the importance of medical knowledge, both theoretical and practical, on the inevitable mistakes that even good physicians make, on the preferability of trusting nature rather than a mediocre doctor, and on the unhappy quarrels that often accompany consultation. He cites the ethical aphorisms of many physicians, including the words of Hippocrates, "be of benefit and do no harm," with Galen's gloss, expressing astonishment that so obvious a rule should need emphasis. Maimonides, however, recalls his own days as a medical student, when he saw many renowned physicians prescribe wrongly. He concludes his reflections with the thought, "There is a general rule, and I have seen great physicians acting on it, that the physician should not treat the disease but the patient who is suffering from it." In a commentary on the First Aphorism of Hippocrates, he insists that a physician must not only diagnose and treat the patient but also provide for patients who cannot afford to buy drugs or pay for an appropriate place of healing, "since these externals are necessary for the attainment of the goal which the physician desires for the patient."[34] Although the detailed medical ethics of the rabbinic commentators did not enter the Western tradition of medical ethics, Jewish respect for the sanctity of life was compatible with Christian belief (indeed, may have surpassed it). The medical historian David Reisman writes, "in a day when the poisoning of rivals and enemies was common, the Jews were the most trustworthy medical advisers".[35]

Beyond this trustworthiness, Jewish physicians acquired a reputation for knowledge and competence. This posed a moral problem for Christian Europe. Enmity toward Jews prompted restrictive measures against Jewish physicians. Church councils passed laws forbidding Christians to visit Jewish doctors but, although these restrictive canons were on the books, they were ignored by those who appreciated good doctors and could afford them, notably the rulers, the nobility, and the Church hierarchy, including more than a few popes. Pope Martin V (1417–1431), favored Jewish physicians and decreed that they could practice among Christians. Despite this occasional tolerance, however, discrimination was ever present, and as medical teaching became more formalized and practice more professional, Jewish practitioners found themselves often excluded from positions of prominence.[36]

Enriched medical learning followed the Arab conquests in every direction: it flowed across northern Africa and entered Europe through Andalusia and Sicily. In the mid-eleventh century, a medical school was established at Salerno in southern Italy, founded, legend says, by two Christians, a Jew, and a Saracen. The actual progenitor of the school at Salerno, Constantine Africanus, was a Carthaginian Muslim who had become a Benedictine monk of Monte Cassino. He fostered the translation and transmission of the Greek and Arabic medical classics throughout medieval Europe.[37] In the course of the next two centuries, volumes of Galen, Avicenna, Rhazes, and Isaac Israeli lay beside the works of ethics and science of Aristotle and the Neo-Platonists on the lecterns in the universities of Italy and France. Medicine became a university subject equal to theology and law, and acquired a set of standard topics and often cited authorities, a formal mode of exposition, and the inevitable examinations leading to degrees. In this way, literate medicine became scholarly medicine and orthodoxies congealed around the scholarship.

The medical literature produced in the world of the universities was principally commentaries on the newly translated medical authorities of the past, now organized like the innovative scholarship of scholastic theology, which framed problems in terms of logically structured *quaestiones* supported by evidence and authority. This format allowed authors to evaluate arguments, criticize opinions, and proffer original views in a systematic fashion. Many of these volumes of learned medicine included sections concerning the virtues of the good physician. These sections contained the admonitions found in the rediscovered writings of classical medicine and are not dissimilar to the decorum and deontology of the monastic medical texts. However, the influence of the new learning began to appear, together with hints of growing professionalism. A treatise by Guglielmo da Saliceto, professor of medicine at the University of Bologna in the late thirteenth century, opens with a description of the good surgeon, who must be learned in medical theory, skilled in practice, and concerned about his patients. The surgeon is urged to acquire *solemnitas*, a term which equates the doctor's decorum with religious ritual and judicial gravity, particularly when conveying information about painful matters. Solemnity will encourage trust in the good judgment of the bearer of the news. This trust will enhance the "honor and praise, as well as the efficacy and good outcome of the medical activity."[38] *Solemnitas* would become a permanent feature of medical decorum as physicians worked to establish a profession esteemed by the public.

Civil authority slowly reasserted itself in the West after the decay of the Western Roman Empire. By the twelfth century, the Holy Roman Empire held hegemony over much of Europe. One of its most extraordinary rulers, Frederick II, King of Sicily, Holy Roman Emperor (1194–1250), was a man of wide learning. He recognized the scholarship of Salerno, which lay within his realms. In 1140, his predecessor, Roger II of Sicily, had decreed that anyone who wished to practice medicine must be examined by royal officials, "lest the King's subjects incur dangers through the inexperience of physicians." In 1231, Frederick went further. "Mindful of the health of our citizens and of the damage and suffering due to the inexperience of physicians," he included in his statement of general law for his realm, the Constitutions of Melfi, a special decree concerning the education and supervision of physicians. A five-year course of medicine, devoted to the "recognized books of Hippocrates and Galen," preceded by the study of the humanities and followed by one year of supervised practice, was prescribed for all candidates. The faculty of Salerno were given the right and the duty to examine all candidates for licensure. The decree also regulated apothecaries and forbade physicians to enter into business deals with them. In addition, it required free service to the poor and regular visits to the sick. By including "ethical obligations" in the law and by requiring an oath to "faithfully fulfill the requirements of the law," Frederick II's decree contributed significantly to the professionalization of physicians, binding them by public declaration into a group that must acknowledge a duty to serve the public. It is almost certain that Frederick II, a marginally orthodox Christian who was strongly attracted to Islamic culture, drew the provisions of the Constitutions of Melfi from the medical world of Islam. He made a political reality of the ideal Plato had envisioned in *Asklepios politicos*, and he encouraged for the first time the politic ethics of medicine that was to grow steadily during the ensuing centuries.[39]

Politic ethics was also fostered by the guilds, unique social institutions that flourished across Europe from the tenth to the fifteenth centuries. Merchants and craftsmen banded together in cities for mutual benefit, and in time created powerful organizations that not only controlled trade and tariffs but also set the conditions of labor, influenced local governance, and provided many services, such as policing and sanitation. These guilds had a strong religious tone, each with its patron saint and its acceptance of duties to provide for the poor and support the Church. They also set standards for the moral behavior of their members. The guilds were the seedbed of the professions. It was to be expected that, as furriers, farriers, and fishmongers achieved fraternal unity and economic power by guilding together, physicians would do so as well. Since the more educated physicians were often associated with the universities, the surgeons and barbers were first to form craft guilds. The Parisian Confraternity of Saints Cosmas and Damien, patron saints of surgeons, was apparently formed in the early thirteenth century; Venetian physicians and surgeons established a guild in 1258; Florentine physicians organized their guild in 1296. Soon even university-trained physicians formed their own collegia, modeled on guilds. The medicosurgical guilds and collegia interacted in complex ways with the university faculties, often disputing the control and licensure of physicians. In 1271, the faculty of the University of Paris issued statutes strictly dividing the responsibilities of physicians, surgeons, and apothecaries, whose roles were differentiated in relation to their mastery of the *scientia medicinae* acquired within the university's halls. The faculty itself had no power to enforce these statutes, but they did persuade civic and church authorities to agree with them in principle (Pope John XXII, who had studied medicine at the University of Paris, particularly favored his old school).[40]

One historian writes, "The foundational principles of medieval medicosurgical guild ethics were that each guild member must (1) be ready to help each other; (2) to protect the well-being and honor of the guild; and (3) to help the sick . . . the guilds were inherently selfish organizations designed to promote the members' special interests."[41] Even though self-interest was at the heart of every guild's organizational life, good works were an essential part of every guild's activities (good works contributed to salvation, which was definitely in one's own interest). For corporations of physicians and surgeons, good works played an even more important part. Physicians' guilds were concerned about the medical qualifications of their membership; about public health measures; about prevention of negligence, malpractice, and quackery; and about the maintenance of fair fees and medical care for the poor. The surgeons of the Confraternity of Saints Cosmas and Damien were reminded of their duties to the poor each time they prayed for the intercession of their patron saints, two third-century physicians revered for their devoted and gratuitous service to the impoverished. Their medieval devotees had to balance that holy obligation against their desire to make a good living. Thus, guild medicine fostered the politic ethics that was later to become so important in medical ethics: good service to city and citizens in return for a monopoly of practice and public prestige. It reinforced an often paradoxical duality between self-interest and altruism at the heart of medical ethics. While Hippocratic physicians may have felt in their hearts the tug between profit and service, that tug was now built into a social organization within which medieval physicians lived and worked. The politic ethics of the profession that was coming into being was, in part, an attempt to reconcile these centrifugal moral impulses and, in part, a somewhat transparent disguise for professional self-interest.[42]

From antiquity on, a *locus classicus* for reflection on the nature, importance, and moral seriousness of the work of medicine was the First Aphorism of Hippocrates. This short text, possibly from Hippocrates' own lips, reads, "Life is short, the art is long, opportunity fleeting, experiment treacherous, judgment difficult. The physician must be ready, not only to do his duty [*deonta*] himself, but also to secure the co-operation of the patient, of the attendants, and of externals [*exothen*]."[43] Galen and many other medical authors found in these enigmatic words room for many thoughts: the intrinsic uncertainty of diagnosis and treatment, the changing nature of disease, the risk of error, and the great responsibility laid upon those who undertake the practice of medicine. Arnau de Vilanova (d. 1311), a Catalan physician who rose to distinction as a professor at Montpellier, wrote several treatises on the First Aphorism of Hippocrates. Vilanova finds in the first phrases four essential points: become expert in the classical literature, go beyond transmitted teachings by careful therapeutic experimentation, draw judicious conclusions about these experiments, and communicate these conclusions with succinct clarity. This advice reflects the scholastic environment of medical learning: logical, critical analysis and exposition of received opinion, together with the medical exigencies of diagnosis, treatment, and communication. The physician's duty in this era of vastly expanded medical knowledge is competence in all these activities, demonstrated not only by a thorough knowledge of medical literature and practical experience but also by a thorough knowledge of the patient, his or her personality, physical state, and social setting. When the physician demonstrates this competence, the cooperation and confidence of patients and others will be won. The final words of the aphorism, the obscure "externals," become for Vilanova the social and economic structure of the relationship between the competent doctor and his patients. Included in this relationship is the matter of *emolumentum*, or payment for services. Appropriate compensation is an intrinsic part of the work of medicine because the patient who pays recognizes the worth of the physician's work. For the patient who cannot pay, the physician's charity also engenders confidence. Thus, all the activities of a skilled physician win merit because they are done out of love, a merit that comes "from God as grace and from man as emolument." Vilanova does not dwell only in the high realms of ethical exhortation. He descends, in another treatise, to a very practical problem of clinical ethics: how best to deal with patients and their relatives who attempt to deceive the physician by presenting false urine specimens for his diagnosis. Although he recommends using a bedside manner that will enhance the patient's trust in the physician's ability, his respect for the truth matches that of those who would deceive him: if you don't understand the case, "say the patient has an obstruction of the liver—particularly using the word 'obstruction' because they do not understand what it means, and it helps greatly that a term is not understood by the people."[44]

An esteemed physician and surgeon in service to three popes, Guy de Chauliac (1290–1370), sums up the medical decorum and deontology commonly found in the literature of learned medieval medicine. His words reflect the new respect for scholarly medicine. A good physician, he says, must not only have extensive experience but also be deeply learned in the theory of medicine, based on *physica*, the natural philosophy of Aristotle (it is about that time that the word *physicus*, or *physician*, became synonymous with the traditional *medicus*). De Chauliac then catalogues the traditional decorum: "The doctor should be well mannered, bold yet cautious, and should abhor false cures or practices. He should be affable to the sick, kindhearted to his colleagues, and wise in his prognostications. He should be chaste, sober, compassionate and merciful. He should not be covetous, grasping in money matters, and then he will receive a fee commensurate with his labors, the financial ability of his patients, the success of the treatment, and his own dignity."[45] De Chauliac, probably quite unconsciously, listed the qualities that the medical profession, then in its nascent stages, would offer as its rationale for a good living: physicians acquire standing in society (dignity) based on manifestly beneficial treatment and thus deserve their fees. During the fifteenth and sixteenth centuries, these qualities would assume more institutional forms. But before traveling there, this history must visit two ancient cultures that had existed outside the ken of the West for many centuries.

3

Medical Ethics of India and China

Literate medicine emerged from folk healing in the cultures of the Occident and the Orient almost simultaneously. In about the fifth century BCE, writings describing disease, its causes, and its remedies appeared in India and China, as well as in the Greek societies of the eastern Mediterranean. This literate medicine also bore the marks of the moral ambiance with which healing is surrounded. In the Occident and the Orient alike, the moral ambiance of that era was shaped by compelling narratives about the origins and meaning of nature and of human life that were created worldwide during the 500 years before the common era. The Vedas of Hindu religion had assumed standard oral forms. The enlightened teachings of the Buddha won adherents in India and Southeast Asia. The social philosophy of Confucius took hold in China. The prophetic poetry of Isaiah and the preaching of Jesus created the matrix of a monotheistic faith that gradually submerged the pagan beliefs of Asia Minor, the Hellenistic world, and the Roman Mediterranean. Literate medicine everywhere was conceived within the visions of these great teachings at both the metaphysical and the moral levels. The medical ethics that developed in India and China paralleled the long tradition in the West. There are remarkable similarities that suggest deeper reflection on how healing and moral meaning are related wherever they are found. There are also major differences that show how much moral belief can affect the form of medicine.

Miracles, magic, and medicine are mixed with morality in the earliest stories of healing, whether related in the Homeric epics, the Vedas of ancient India, or the writings from the feudal states that preceded the great dynasties of China. Almost at the same time that the Greek Pindar sang of Asklepios, the "peerless physician," an Indo-Aryan poet fashioned in Sanskrit an analogous legend about the beginnings of medicine. Twin "sons of the Sun," the Ashvini, are called "physicians of the gods," and are masters of healing using incantation and herbs. The Ashvini learned the secrets of healing from a sage to whom Indra, god of storms, had imparted them under a vow of secrecy. They enticed the sage to teach them his secrets and, endowed with this new knowledge, disguised the sage to protect him from the angry god by a zenotransplant, replacing his head with the head of a horse. This deception was futile. Says an historian of Indian medicine, "Some of the more fastidious gods took exception to this mode of learning. . . . Cutting off one's preceptor's head, though with the best of intentions, was denounced as an atrocious act and the Ashvini were outcast by the gods."[1] The twin physicians again used their newfound skills to restore the virility of a newly married but decrepit sage, who succeeded in having the outcasts restored to their ritual status. Indra, however, remained angry. He prepared to cast a thunderbolt, but his arm was paralyzed. The Ashvini healed the god and finally attained revered status as premier practitioners of Indian medicine.

In both Greek and Hindu legends medicine comes to humans as divine knowledge, and it must be used in conformity with the divine will that imparted it. Since the divine will is not always communicated in an Olympian decree or a deity's dictate, the morality surrounding healing must be constructed out of the culture's broader moral beliefs. Hindu religion is a rich amalgam of cosmogony, mythology, ritual, and moral injunctions. The Upanishads spread the belief in reincarnation and *karma*, the belief that all actions produce consequences for future life. The believer, by devotion, meritorious action, and asceticism, liberates himself from mundane existence and readies himself for reincarnation in a better form and finally, in achievement of oneness between the individual soul (*atman*) and the universal being (*brahman*). The *dharma* or "right path" to salvation is expressed with particular clarity in the *Law of Primordial Man* (*Manu-Smrti*). The first section of this book presents a Hindu analogue of the Judeo-Christian decalogue, forbidding evil in thought, word and deed, such as coveting the property of others, abusing them, lying, slander and sexual intercourse with a woman married to another man. These general injunctions are followed by particular rules appropriate to the pure life of the priestly Brahmans, the rigorous life of the ascetic Sadhus, the duties of women and the justice required of rulers. All persons are admonished to give pain to no creature and, by performing their duties and avoiding sin, to accumulate spiritual merit for their reincarnation. Truthfulness, in particular, is praised as the unequaled means of purification of the soul and the most efficacious form of austerity. Hindu life imposes a rigorous morality on its faithful.[2]

Even in its practical aspects, Indian medicine is rooted in the sacred, the ritual, and the moral.[3] One of the Vedic scriptures, *Atharva Veda*, consists of charms, hymns, and incantations to ward off disease, describing healing as a shamanic, magical activity. However, another form of healing was emerging from the experience of wandering ascetics (*sramanas*) who employed herbal medicines, ointments, and various therapeutic diets. These healers slowly formulated a pharmacopoeia and a rudimentary theory of disease causation. Theory and skills evolved into a "science of life" (*ayurveda*). Although it appears that the original practitioners of *ayurveda* were cast out of orthodox Brahman society, both because they mingled with the common people and because they preferred their empirical, practical knowledge to the esoteric priestly wisdom, eventually *ayurveda* was incorporated into Hindu orthodoxy.[4] Two classical Sanskrit works, *Caraka Samhita* and *Susruta Samhita*, composed around the beginning of the common era, are the Indian parallels to the Hippocratic Collection in the Western world. Attributed to two semilegendary physicians, Agnivesa and Susruta, these works elaborate a theory of physiology and disease, as well as a practical therapeutics within a general Hindic worldview. These and other ancient texts contain the essence of ayurvedic medicine: treatises on drugs and surgery, treatment of children's diseases, antidotes for poison, and restoration of vigor and virility. These texts place the work of healing within a philosophy of life that is thoroughly Brahman.

Humans are a microcosm in constant flux with the macrocosm whose elements of fire, wind, and water constitute the physical body and whose divine origins arise from chaos and flow into multiple forms of matter and spirit. Health is a balance of the *doshas* or humors—*wind, bile,* and *phlegm*—words whose English translation impoverishes these complex metaphysical and physiological concepts. Balance is maintained by all sorts of conscious and unconscious interactions between the person and the physical, religious, and social environments. Not only do food, weather, and hygiene affect health; psychological attitudes and social experiences also affect the humoral balance. Inherent qualities of goodness, vitality, and inertia are present in all substances and are manifested in food, activity, and moral character. The work of the physician contributes to the moral purpose toward which all persons must aim: to transform physical and mental dispositions from the lowest state of inertia to the highest virtues of spiritual knowledge and attainment. Medicine consists in discovering how the organic unity within and without the body has become fragmented; the *vaidya* or physician "takes apart the bodily components, cleanses them, and puts them back together." This is done in the service of organic and spiritual liberation.

It is not surprising, in a religion so imbued with moral precepts and a medicine in which body and spirit are so closely integrated, that a medical treatise should also set out the *dharma* for patients and practitioners alike. Both of the classical treatises list the ethical qualities that contribute to the wholeness and health of all persons and therefore are necessary for those who would engage in healing. All persons must respect the gods, cows, Brahmans, teachers, and the elderly and observe religous rites; all should be scrupulously clean and "friendly to all creatures, reconcile the angry, console the frightened, be merciful to the poor, be predominantly of compromising nature and tolerant toward others, never tell a lie or take others' property or long for others' wives or disclose secrets." Good physicians must follow all these precepts and, in addition, have deep knowledge of medical science and practical skills in its application. They must "nurture cordial feelings exactly like the mother, father and kin to all creatures. . . . Physicians with such qualities give life to patients and cure their diseases." In one moral matter, physicians are given special license: they may tell a lie in order to save the life of the patient. Unfortunately, there are many pseudophysicians, "the worst among idiots who undertake medicine only to earn a livelihood." They loudly proclaim their skills but hide themselves from the questions of the learned. They ensnare the sick by their specious manners and then abandon them when problems occur. "These are the messengers of death on earth; hence they should be boycotted."[5] *Susruta Samhita* contains similar descriptions of the physician's character and duties, and insists that the physician must not only be intelligent and resolute but also respect truth (*satya*) and duty (*dharma*) as the most sacred principles of life.

Caraka Samhita also contains an oath, possibly intended to be sworn by initiates in medicine. The first injunction of this oath recalls the Oath of Hippocrates but surpasses it in eloquence and moral idealism. The Hippocratic words are, "I will apply treatment for the benefit of the sick according to my ability and judgment; I will keep them from harm and injustice." *Caraka* says, "Day and night, however you may be engaged, you shall strive for the relief of the patient with all your heart and soul. You shall not desert or injure your patient even for the sake of your life or living." The physician is also enjoined to enter the patient's house only with permission and in company with someone known to the patient and to keep private "the peculiar customs of the patient's household" to which he has been admitted. Women should be respected and never seduced. The physician must study diligently and attain knowledge of his art from every reliable source. It is not suitable to speak of a patient's approaching death, nor should a physician attempt to treat a disease known to be fatal. In addition to these deontological precepts, the physician is urged to be clean, modest in dress, polite, and truthful in speech, as well as to avoid boastful words, quarrels, and arguments. In striking contrast to the Judeo-Christian tradition, the Oath of Caraka warns physicians not to treat enemies of the king or outlaws.[6]

Although *ayurveda* may have begun among the ascetics who accepted no reward for their healing work, Hindu physicians may earn a good living, but they should treat patients without regard for personal gain. Although Hindu religion advises no one to approach his ruler, his teacher, or his physician without a gift, the physician should not expect a poor person to make an offering. Those who can pay but do not are considered wicked. The physician's dutiful treatment of patients wins religious merit for his next life. In general, the work of a physician fulfills the three main purposes of life revealed in the Upanishads: religious duty, attainment of pleasure, and achievement of wealth. The physician's care of the sick relieves suffering and adds to human happiness, thus fulfilling his religious duty; the satisfaction of reputation and the gratitude of those whom he has healed contributes to pleasure; and the achievement of wealth is the legitimate return for his service to wealthy patients. Thus, the physician's work fits within his religious life.

Vedic religion designates three social classes rigorously divided from each other: the priestly class of Brahmans; the secular ruling class of Ksatriyas; and the artisans, herders and farmers, the Vaisyes. Below these three classes are the Shudras, who served the upper classes, and the impure or untouchables. These classes are diversified into many castes by origin, occupation, and religious practices. The relation of these castes to one another is defined by innumerable rules, violation of which involves spiritual pollution. Although early Vedic texts prohibit Brahmans from practicing medicine, men from every caste, from Brahmans to Shudras, were eventually allowed to become physicians, although the rules of ritual purity limited the kinds of behavior allowed to Brahman physicians, who could not come into contact with the dead or with bodily excretions. However, physicians from one class could not treat the sick who belonged to a class or caste with which interaction was prohibited. Practitioners of medicine eventually formed a unique caste in which medical knowledge was passed through families. The rigorous laws of ritual purity, however, made it difficult for physicians to demonstrate universal concern. As one author remarks after praising the spirituality and high moral standards of Hindu life, "Doubtless, Hinduism lacks something of that spirit of charity which abounds in Buddhism. . . . In his concern for purity, the Hindu tends rather to keep aloof than to give himself."[7]

Buddhist medicine presents a striking contrast to the caste discrimination of Hindu medicine. In the sixth century BCE, Siddartha Gautama, a prince of Nepal, gave the world a faith, known to its adherents as *Sasana* or the Teaching (about achieving wisdom and virtue) and known to the world as Buddhism after Gautama became the Buddha or Enlightened One. In his lifetime, the Buddha realized, first through asceticism and then through meditation, the great Truth that human life is suffering due to the changing nature of material life, that suffering could be transcended by understanding, and that liberation from the suffering of life could be achieved by right thought and right deeds. After his death, the doctrine of the eightfold path of enlightenment, whereby humans could transcend the suffering of material, mutable existence, won adherents throughout India and Asia.

Medicine was part of Buddhist life from its earliest days. Although all life is suffering, compassion for the sufferer is Buddhism's highest virtue. The Buddha himself is frequently called the "Great Physician." Among the four sublime virtues that all Buddhists should cultivate on the path to enlightenment is compassion, the desire to relieve the sufferings of all other living things. Particularly in Mahayanist Buddhism, wisdom and duty summon even *bodhisattvas*, enlightened persons who have achieved perfection, to delay their reward in order to relieve suffering humankind. This teaching, which encouraged a life of compassionate benevolence toward others rather than a hermetic removal from society, counted care for the sick as a prime value. It is told that Gautama once encountered a dying monk who had been ignored by his brethren, who were intent on their own salvation. The Buddha himself nursed the sick monk and admonished them, "You,

O monks, have neither a mother nor a father who could nurse you. If, O monks, you do not nurse one another, who will nurse you? Whoever, O monks, would nurse me, he should nurse the sick."[8] The same scripture describes the duties of those who care for the sick, instructing them to assuage their brother's pain by attendance, motivated by kindly thoughts rather than greed, willingness to undertake even disgusting tasks, recitation of prayers, and cheering the sick one in his final hours. In accord with this teaching, the monastic community (*sangha*) established a regimen for the care of sick monks and welcomed all in need of medical aid. Unlike the caste-bound Hindus, Buddhists could mix with all people without fear of ritual contamination. The science of ayurvedic medicine became the practice of Buddhist medicine, which easily crossed all caste lines and was not limited by rigorous laws of ritual purity that limited Hindu *vaidyas*. After the conversion of King Asoka in the third century BCE, hospitals served by monks were established throughout the Indian realms under his rule. Within the first 500 years of the common era, Buddhist missionaries brought the teaching of the Buddha and the practice of compassionate care for the sick into China, Southeast Asia, Tibet, Korea, and Japan.[9]

China has its own rich medical history that antedates the arrival of Buddhist forms of ayurvedic medicine.[10] Healing techniques in which magical incantations and medicinal herbs are marshaled against demon-induced diseases appear in the earliest evidence of Chinese culture. During the Han dynasties (−206 to +220), the Chinese Empire assumed the essential shape it was to maintain until the first decade of the twentieth century. Under the hegemony of the emperor, a vast bureaucracy managed every aspect of public life. Entry into the bureaucracy was limited to those educated in the Confucian classics. The social and political thought of Confucius (−552 to −479) became paramount. A wandering teacher of minor princes, he prized orderly administration of the state, bringing peace and welfare to all its people. This was to be achieved by assiduous observance of rites and a morality of respect toward one's parents, elders, colleagues, and rulers. A rich panoply of virtues, led by *ren*, love of humanity, must inform the life of the good man (*junzi*), all aimed at creating harmony between personal and social life, called the Way (*Tao*). *The Analects*, a book composed by the first disciples of Confucius, opens with the words "A man who respects his parents and his elders would hardly be inclined to defy his superiors. A man who is not inclined to defy his superiors will never foment a rebellion. A gentleman [*junzi*] works at the root. Once the root is secured, the Way [*Tao*] unfolds. To respect parents and elders is the root of humanity [*ren*]."[11] The Han rulers adopted the wisdom of Confucius, who had been dead for several centuries, as the philosophy of their state.

During those years, philosophical views about nature and society began to emerge from common beliefs, within which a comprehensive medicine developed. A doctrine of nature that saw all phenomena as the product of dynamic and cyclic forces, named *yin* and *yang*, provided an explanation for disease, as did the parallel doctrine of the Five Phases, the ever-changing correspondence between the primordial elements, designated as water, wood, fire, metal, and soil. Health and disease are disorders of excess and deficiency in the patterns of these forces and elements. This physiological theory fostered a way of healing that moved beyond the magical and shamanistic practices of antiquity, although it never entirely banished them.

These ideas found classic expression in *Nei Jing* (*The Yellow Emperor's Classic of Inner Medicine*), the Chinese analogue to the Hippocratic Collection and the Indian *Samhitas*. Like these works, it is a collection of medical texts, possibly dating from the second century BCE. Unity is imposed on these heterogeneous texts by the questions posed by a legendary ruler, Huang Di, to a "divinely inspired teacher," Tianshi, about longevity, the causes of health and disease, and the diagnosis and treatment of various illnesses. The general outlines of traditional Chinese medicine appear in these dialogues: the *yin/yang* theory, an imaginative anatomy and physiology of vital energy (*qi*), the application of pulse diagnosis, and the therapies of acupuncture and moxibustion (relatively little is said about herbal pharmacotherapy, which later becomes a major feature of Chinese therapeutics) and provides an elaborate schema relating *Yin/Yang*, the Five Phases, and the seasonal changes to the health of the body and spirit.[12]

Although the *yin/yang* and Five Phases doctrines are described in physical and cosmological terms, they are profoundly rooted in moral and social conceptions. A modern translator of *Nei Jing* comments that it is not merely a medical textbook: it is a "treatise on general ethics and regimen of life, including the prevailing Chinese religious beliefs." The dialogues open with the emperor's question, "Why did the men of former times live past 100 years?" The teacher answers, "Because they understood the *Tao* (the divinely ordained order of nature and life), patterned their lives on the *yin/yang* . . . lived temperate, orderly lives . . . exercising restraint of will and desire, kept their hearts pure, at peace and without fear and were not misled by excess and evil."[13] The association between virtue and health is a constant theme in the dialogues. Similarly, the association between personal virtue and social order is emphasized. The Chinese concern about social order and harmony, developed to its acme in the teachings of Confucius, penetrates the fundamental conceptions of health, disease, and medicine. Book III of *Nei Jing*, for example, describes the human anatomy in terms of the roles of various public officials who serve the emperor in maintaining a sound society. When the monarch himself is intelligent and enlightened, the society is peaceful and thriving; similarly, health arises from harmony within the body, each function and organ properly related to others. Another passage declares, "The sages do not treat those who have already fallen ill but rather those who are not yet ill. They do not put the state in order only when revolt is underway but before an insurrection occurs."[14] It is the duty of the physician to know how to preserve the order of the body and, if it is disrupted, how to return it to order. This is not merely a metaphor: social health was profoundly linked with personal health, and personal health came from a regular life, following moral and ritual rules and, above all, manifesting righteousness, humaneness, and compassion. The right practice of medicine is impossible unless it is connected with the right governance of society: "[doctors] discuss the diseases until they advance to the origins of the government; they treat the diseases with a knowledge which equals that of public administration." The ills of the physical body occur in conjunction with the changes of *yin/yang* in heaven and on earth: the knowledge of the good physician must encompass all "Confucian scholarship" (*ru*), the "scientific insight into heaven, earth and man."[15] A medieval commentator on the *Nei Jing* states that the Emperor Huang Di ruled his empire by the principle that "the body is connected with all the rest."[16]

The physiological and medical doctrines of *Nei Jing* were formed within two dominant cultural philosophies, Confucianism and Taoism. Both of these views, formulated by the sages Confucius and Laozi in the fourth century BCE, provided theoretical explanations and metaphors within which observed states of disease and health and the factors influencing them could be situated. The influence of Confucian social and moral philosophy has been noted. The influence of Taoism bears more immediately on the physical aspects of medicine. The teachings of Laozi and his followers emphasized the absolute and universal reality, to which human understanding and living must conform. This reality was given the name *Tao*, the same word that, in Confucian thought refers to the moral path of individuals in society but that in Taoism embraces the more metaphysical principle of universal nature. *The Book of Nature and Intelligence*, attributed to Laozi, begins, "It is Nature itself [*Tao*], and not any part abstracted from Nature, which is the ultimate source of all that happens, all that comes and goes, all that begins and ends, is and is not." This *Tao* is revealed in all the workings of the natural world and has moral implications: "Intelligence (*De*) consists in acting according to Nature (*Tao*). . . . Nature sustains itself through three precious principles, which one does well to embrace and follow: gentleness, frugality and humility."[17] Taoist scholars encouraged knowledge of natural processes of every sort, and both contemplation and scientific study were prized. Longevity and even immortality were sought and earned by a life of simplicity and tranquility. The power of nature to contribute to longevity was exploited by both magic and pharmacology. Much of the impetus toward the creation of an elaborate pharmacopoeia for Chinese medicine came from Taoism. Taoist monks engaged in both ritualistic and medical healing.

A third worldview entered the history of Chinese medicine when Buddhism entered China in the first century CE. The monks brought not only the *dharma* but also knowledge of medicine, fundamentally rooted in Vedic science but modified by many Buddhist notions. Ancient texts frequently mix Vedic notions of physiology with Buddhist notions of morality: "three grave sicknesses of the body are of wind, heat and cold, healed by various medications; three grave illness of humankind are anger, desire and ignorance and these are healed by compassion and meditation."[18] Buddhism, which was first perceived in China as a variant of Taoism, spread widely as a faith of the common people and also achieved respectability among the intellectuals. As in India, its monks provided medical aid to all in need and established hospitals and dispensaries. The central ethical notions of Buddhism mingled with Confucian ideas and were indelibly imprinted on Chinese medical thought. The primary virtue of Buddhism, compassion (*ci*), and the primary precept of Confucianism, humaneness (*ren*), are constant reminders to those who would be "great" or "enlightened" physicians (*da yi, ming yi*).[19]

Confucian teaching not only provided a theory and a language for medical understanding, it also affected the social organization of medicine. Preeminent in Confucian ethics is the reverence for parents and duties toward the family. These duties included maintenance of the health of one's parents and family; thus, knowledge of medicine was necessary for all good sons, and its practice was directed primarily to one's own family. Said one medical writer, "Knowledge of medicine is indispensable in the assistance of one's relatives. All the renowned physicians of former times . . . started to practice medicine because their mothers fell ill."[20] Also, Confucian thought discouraged the fostering of specialists in different aspects of life. The Confucian scholar was uniformly learned in the classics and adept at all skills needed for social life, from military leadership to medicine. Thus, the formation of a distinct profession of physicians was discouraged; indeed, the term *physician* (*yi*) was somewhat demeaning. Nevertheless, scholars who had especially deep knowledge of the medical classics and particular skill in their application sometimes cared for persons outside their families and attained a reputation as "enlightened physicians." Many of these scholars became full-time practitioners, although often within the official ranks of the elaborate imperial court system. As civil servants who had passed the rigorous examinations in the classics, they were often given the title "Confucian physicians" (*ru yi*).

There were also persons who, although not classical scholars, were well read in the medical literature and who dared to practice medicine to make a living. These "common physicians" (*rong yi*) were derisively called *bell doctors*, for they advertised themselves by walking through the streets ringing a bell. Finally, many others engaged in the healing arts, whom the scholarly doctors branded as sorcerer-doctors (*wu yi*). These distinctions persisted throughout Chinese history, and constant debates discussed the merits of various sorts of practice. As a result, while medicine and certain classes of practitioners were held in high esteem, no cohesive, independent profession of medicine ever emerged in Chinese society, as it did in the West. Even "enlightened physicians" considered themselves Confucian classical scholars, rather than medical practitioners, and owed their professional allegiance to the imperial bureaucracy within which most of them worked. As Paul

Unshuld, a historian of Chinese medicine, says, "To organize this elite group would have been a logical step, and in the West it was carried out. . . . Yet in the Confucian society this did not happen."[21]

The apogee of classical Chinese medicine came in the seventh century of the common era, during the splendid Tang dynasty (+618 to 905). A large medical literature and a wide variety of therapeutics had matured over the previous centuries. The Three Great Teachings—Confucianism, Taoism, and Buddhism—had thoroughly penetrated medical thinking. Medical education had been initiated in the venerable Imperial University (founded in the first century BCE), and medical officers had been appointed in the imperial bureaucracy. An official pharmacopoeia was compiled, and standard editions of classical medical books were published. Around the year +845, Buddhism fell into disfavor in official circles, being seen as a foreign import that threatened Chinese ideas and institutions.[22] Monasteries were suppressed, and the number of Buddhist charitable institutions shrank. Hospitals and hospices, orphanages, and infirmaries that had been served by Buddhist monks and nuns were brought under government administration (it is interesting to note that the Buddhist hospices, called *Compassionate Pastures*, were renamed *Patients' Compounds* by the bureaucrats). When, after a century of disfavor, Buddhism was again welcomed in imperial circles, the monks and nuns returned to their charitable work, but government control was maintained. The National Medical Administration was strengthened to oversee these institutions and provide public health measures. Certifying examinations were set for admission and promotion as a "great" or "Confucian" physician, and it is possible that the examination system found its way into the West from China.[23] An Imperial Medical College with designated professorships and a curriculum was established, and provincial colleges of similar form were created in every administrative district. Cities of certain sizes were required to have specific numbers of medical students (e.g., 100,000 families = 20 medical students). An Arabic traveler in China during that time noted that medical prescriptions were posted on public signboards so that the common people could read them. In addition, considerable contact with Arabic, ayurvedic, and Nestorian Christian medical scientists was fostered, and medical missions traveled from China to Japan, Korea, and other neighboring nations.

During that golden era of Chinese medicine the first major writing on the ethics of medicine appeared, coming, strangely enough, from a common physician. Sun Simiao (+581 to +682) learned medicine, it is said, to support his own fragile health and became a physician of great renown, called the "King of Prescriptions." Although invited by three successive emperors to become a court physician, he declined and continued to practice in a rural village. He was a scholar equally committed to each of the Three Great Teachings, and he drew from each elements of his medical ethics. At the beginning of his vast treatise on pharmacological and magical medicine, *Qianjin fang* (*Prescriptions of the Thousand Ounces of Gold*),

Sun Simiao describes "the absolute sincerity of the Great Physician." Such a physician approaches the patient with utmost attention and concentration on the signs of the disease, having mastered the fundamentals of medicine. When he treats the patient, he must be mentally calm and compassionate in disposition, "committing himself firmly to the willingness to take the effort to save every living creature."

There follows a passage that ranks high as an ethical credo for physicians in any culture. It is written in words that are clearly Buddhist in inspiration.

> If someone seeks help because of illness . . . a Great Physician should not pay attention to status, wealth or age, neither should he question whether the person is attractive or unattractive, whether he is an enemy or a friend, whether he is Chinese or a foreigner, or finally whether he is uneducated or educated. He should meet everyone on equal ground; he should always act as if he were thinking of himself. . . . Neither dangerous mountain passes nor the time of day, neither weather conditions nor hunger, thirst or fatigue should keep him from helping whole-heartedly.

Sun Simiao goes on to extol the Buddhist virtue of compassion, which should extend to animals as well as humankind and which urges the treatment of even the most repugnant illnesses. He then describes the decorum for physicians: they must speak in a polite manner, not be impressed by wealth, and not indulge in fine food and drink in the houses of patients. Above all, they should not be conceited about their skills: "someone who has accidentally healed a disease, stalks about with his head raised, shows conceit and announces that no one in the entire world could measure up to him." The author then sighs, saying with knowing resignation, "In this respect all physicians are evidently incurable." He then refers to the doctrine of the second "great teaching," Taoism. Laozi taught that good deeds are rewarded by the spirits and evil punished by them; in comparison to these rewards and punishments, human praise and retribution are trivial. Physicians should then develop attitudes of goodwill, compassion, and magnanimity, moving on the right path even when concealed from human eyes. Neither reputation nor wealth should be the object: "the object is to help [the sick]." As an example, the author admonishes that "the wealth [of the patient] should not be the reason to prescribe precious and expensive drugs and thus make access to help more difficult and underscore one's merits and abilities."[24]

About 150 years after this compendium of medical ethics appeared, Lu Zhi, a high-ranking Confucian physician in the imperial court reinforced the prejudice against the practice of medicine for profit. Lu Zhi's short treatise develops the Confucian theme that "medicine is practiced humaneness" (*ren shu*). The quality of humaneness, according to Mencius, the first great commentator on Confucius, is innate in all humans, but it must be drawn forth by education and practice. For physicians, this means the willingness to hasten to relieve the sufferer and to do so without thought for one's own profit, reputation, or the accumulation of wealth for one's children. The physician who "plans for profit" should be "considered a thief."[25] Another Confucian physician, Kou Zongshi, presented a pragmatic

rationale for the virtue of physicians: "when the physician is not guided by compassion and humaneness, the patient begins to doubt and despise the physician."[26]
Jiang Chou, a thirteenth-century Confucian physician, wrote an appealing treatise, *Yigong baoying* (*Retributions for Medical Services*), consisting of twelve short
stories about good and bad physicians. Good physicians treat persons in need with
effective medicine, show generosity toward those unable to pay, and, in two stories,
reject sexual rewards for their services. Bad physicians use fraudulent remedies,
are greedy, and neglect their patients. (One story is not about a physician but about
the torments inflicted by heaven on a woman who was an abortionist.) Good physicians are rewarded with long life and success in their practice, the praise of
others, and good fortune; bad ones are punished by disaster in life and demonic
beatings after death. The maxim "When another person is ill, it is as though I myself
am ill" is extolled and exemplified by a good physician who "practiced medicine
without ever speaking of money." His reward was the preservation by the gods of
his house and cattle when fire destroyed his town.[27] Certainly, many physicians
fell short of these high ideals, as noted in the treatise of a seventeenth-century
scholarly physician, Gong Tingxian, whose words are memorable: "In former
times, the principles of medicine . . . were applied with the aim of keeping men
alive. Yet many physicians nowadays do not know this old significance. When
they visit the rich, they are conscientious; when they deal with the poor, they act
carelessly. This is the eternal peculiarity of those who practice medicine as a
profession. . . . Medicine is responsibility over life and death . . . [and all who
practice it] should adopt the highest virtue, love of life."[28]

Down through the centuries, these themes are repeated in many treatises on
medical ethics. The physician must be learned and skilled, generous and compassionate, continent and restrained, courteous and courtly, and attentive to the needs
of rich and poor, noble and commoner. The moral values of Buddhism and Confucianism—above all, humaneness and compassion—are always invoked. An
early-nineteenth-century treatise, *Yi-zhen* (*Warnings for Physicians*), by Huai Yuan
expresses this thesis beautifully: "In medical practice one cannot act at one's own
discretion. Patients entrust physicians with the decision over their death, and our
own responsibility is based on the principle of requital later on. . . . In its origin
medicine is applied humaneness. To see other people suffer arouses compassion
and pity within oneself. Their hope and trust are infinite. Who should help them,
if not I?"[29]

In the sixteenth century, Western medicine reached China and India when Jesuit
missionaries entered the Middle Kingdom and Portuguese traders settled at Goa.
One Jesuit, Claudius Visdelou, successfully treated the malaria of Emperor Kangxi
with quinine ("Jesuit bark") in 1693. However, the medical treatises introduced by
Europeans were treated as curiosities by both Chinese and Indian medical scholars, and this incursion of post-Galenic, premodern medicine was not broadly influential. However, in the nineteenth century, the British, who dominated the Indian

subcontinent, and American Protestant missions in China introduced the new physiology and microbiology and modest therapies, particularly surgical ones, of the times. In China, particularly after the declaration of the Republic in 1912, Western medicine assumed great prestige, and although traditional practitioners far outnumbered Western-trained ones, government health policy encouraged modern medicine and discouraged traditional practice. One prominent Western-trained Chinese physician repudiated any link with traditional practitioners with the harsh words "why should modern medicine accept this marriage proposal from such a lazy, stupid wife with bound feet wrapped in yards of smelly bandages."[30] It was not until after the proclamation of the People's Republic of China that interest revived in rapprochement between Western and traditional medicine.

With the acculturation of Western medical science came something of Western medical ethics. Yet even the modern physicians realized that, while traditional medicine might lack a scientific basis, Chinese medical ethics is not outmoded. In 1933, Dr. Song Guobin, a Western-trained physician, published *The Ethics of Medical Practice*, in which he tried to integrate Western medical ethics with traditional ethics drawn from Confucianism. Ethics is the *tao*—path or way and, by extension, moral principle—of practicing medicine and consists of the Confucian concepts of humaneness and righteousness. Song defined humaneness by the Western concept of fraternity and defined righteousness as what is appropriately done in compliance with humaneness. Physicians should love people and desire to do good. The physician's responsibility to the patient is to treat disease, promote health, and relieve suffering. The physician should have the virtues of diligence, devotion, warmheartedness, and dignity. The principle of humaneness requires physicians to treat poor patients for free when necessary; the principle of righteousness requires them to be competent, not to do harm, not to take advantage of the patient's vulnerability for their own benefit, not to experiment uselessly, and not to practice favoritism. On the moral character of physicians, Song followed the Chinese tradition, emphasizing the right ordering of one's thoughts and feelings and the right ordering of one's world: the physician who is not himself ordered in body and spirit can hardly order the body and spirit of his patient. Song is the first writer in Chinese medical ethics to argue systematically for the obligation of confidentiality, although he recognized that this obligation is not unconditional. The patient's consent to disclosure, possible harm to others, or the legitimate needs of criminal justice release the physician from confidentiality. Among colleagues, physicians should respect themselves and others, and should maintain a friendly feeling and a modest attitude. The obligation of the physician to the state and society is to prevent disease and death, to apply remedial measures, to investigate the cause of death, and to support public charities. Song rejected contraception and abortion as immoral. His book became a modern classic on the ethics of physician behavior, although its influence was limited largely to the academic world of medicine.[31]

In the literate medicine of ancient and medieval India and China, we can see the analogues of the deontology and decorum we have described in the Western tradition. The Hindu principle of respect for all life and the virtues of honesty, generosity, and hospitality recall the Judeo-Christian reverence for the sanctity of life and the duties of charity that follow from such reverence. The Chinese deontology consists of the Buddhist and Confucian virtues of humaneness and compassion, which parallel the principles of beneficence and nonmaleficence of Hippocratic and Judeo-Christian medicine. The duties of learning and competence follow from these virtues and principles. In addition, a few other duties approach the absolute in both cultures, particularly, the prohibitions of sexual and financial exploitation of patients and their families. The rules of decorum of the Occidental and Oriental traditions are strikingly similar: the physician exhibits an etiquette in manner and in word that will render him gracious to the patient. Certainly, the physician's actual behavior must have differed greatly from society to society. Still, the general intent of this social advice is clear (indeed, there is occasionally remarkably similar counsel: both Hippocrates and Lu Zhi warn physicians to avoid elaborate hairstyles and headgear).[32]

In one important respect, Oriental and Occidental medical ethics are very different: in India and China, there is no politic ethics for the profession, for the simple reason that a profession, in the modern Western sense, never evolved in these cultures. Ayurvedic medicine was caste-bound from the beginning, and the rules of ritual purity provided the ethics of the physician's relations with society. In China, the long debate over the propriety of medical practice outside the family and the receipt of money for service inhibited the development of a profession. The Confucian physicians were professionlike but never had the need to organize themselves into distinctive groups: they were already a distinctive body of civil servants with classical education and court duties. Other practitioners were never able to amass the social power that would support professional organization. Even when there was some state oversight of medical practice, as there was from time to time in ancient India and imperial China, there was never an implicit social contract between a formal profession and the society. Whereas in the West, after the Renaissance, the politic ethics of professional medicine significantly augmented the deontology and decorum of the long tradition, in the East, medical morality remained a deontology, rooted in religious and philosophical beliefs, and a decorum of polite and gracious behaviors.

It is perilous to generalize from such widely disparate social settings and literary sources. Nevertheless, after reading the sources, it is possible to present a tentative generalization. In Occidental and Oriental cultures with a literate medicine, certain ethical precepts and counsel seem to be universally imposed upon those who would practice the healing arts. First, respect life; second, have the requisite knowledge and skills to offer oneself as a healer; third, be compassionate to the sick; fourth, do not seek personal gain at the expense of the sick who seek your help; fifth, be sexually chaste with your patients and their families; sixth, be polite and gentle with your patients; seventh, do not discriminate between rich and poor patients. In neither the East nor the West is there any allusion to the autonomy of the patient. The strictures of confidentiality are suggested only in the warning to refrain from loose talk about the patient's household. Telling the truth to patients is hardly mentioned in any tradition until the nineteenth-century debates among English and American authors (although Book I of *Nei Jing* ends with the enigmatic words "Not to teach [medicine] to the wrong person and never to tell or act a lie is called the achievement of *Tao*").[33] These similarities across very different cultures and era make one wonder whether there may not be some inherent and universal moral atmosphere that surrounds the work of caring for the sick and pervades that work, regardless of culturally diverse moral systems.

4

Renaissance and Enlightenment
Fourteenth to Eighteenth Centuries

European medicine entered the fourteenth century well ensconced in the universities and, to some extent, regulated by civil authorities. Orthodoxies had formed around the classical medical texts and their commentaries. The medical literature was studied side by side with scientific, moral, political, and theological literature. Guilds of physicians had formed, and a nascent profession had appeared. The scholarly physicians, who had "read" medicine and could justify their diagnoses and therapies by reference to a text and a theory were a small island in the sea of semiliterate practitioners, folk healers, and quacks, but on that island the science and ethics of medicine flourished. A fourteenth-century Flemish physician, Jan Yperman, stated that physicians and surgeons "must not only have a knowledge of medicine but must also know the books of nature, which is called philosophy . . . the doctor must also know ethics, as this science teaches good morals."[1]

Medical science slowly grew. The Galenic and Arabic classics that had initiated the medical renaissance of the Middle Ages, and had been organized in the thirteenth and early fourteenth centuries by such authors as John of Arderne, Henri de Mondeville, Guy de Chauliac, and Arnau de Vilanova, were not considered dated when printing presses began to mass-produce scholarly books in the mid-fifteenth century. However, classical and medieval scholarship was quickly advanced by medical scholars embued with the Renaissance hunger for new learning. Authors such as Sanctorius, Fracastoro, Fallopius, Vesalius, and Fabricius contributed to physiological, pathological, and anatomical understanding. Although most of this scholarship remained speculative or at the level of uncritical experience, it gradually moved toward such critical revelations as the experiment-based knowledge of William Harvey (1578–1657) and Marcello Malpighi (1628–1694) concerning the circulation of blood. An odd genius, Theophrastus Philippus Aureolus Bombastus von Hohenheim, known as Paracelsus (1493–1541), challenged the entire Galenic system and opened the way to a new pharmacology. Not only did the science of medicine move in new directions during the Renaissance; the elements of a profession started to emerge, and the politic ethics of medicine became more prominent.

Medical authors still introduced their books on medical theory and practice with the customary treatise on the characteristics of the good doctor. While these authors repeated the classical doctrines of Hippocrates and Galen, as well as the admonitions of the Christian faith, a new element appeared: the importance of competence, defined as mastery of the literature and its reasoned application to the medical problem of the patient. "The specific morality of the practitioner," says a historian of this era, "derived from his being a healer technically trained and was essential for his status as an expert in medicine."[2] In light of this overarching moral imperative, medical authors comment on the problems that will inevitably arise in the relationship with patients: how to ensure the confidence of the patient and compliance with the regimen, how to deal with other physicians who may be involved in the case, and how to define the nature of the contractual relationship with patients and its economic aspects.

This renaissance in medical scholarship was occurring during an era in which Western Europe was also becoming aware of the possibilities of more complex forms of commerce. The emerging profession of scholarly medicine fitted into that world. The financial relationship between physician and patient was increasingly viewed as a commercial transaction determined by certain constant features. For centuries, medical fees had been viewed within the ancient Roman tradition of *honoraria*: those engaged in the learned professions, such as teachers, scribes, and physicians, were paid with a gift determined by the satisfaction of the employer or client. During the Renaissance, another term in Roman law, *salarium*, begins to appear in medical writings about the payment of physicians. A *salarium* is a fixed sum calculated according to the nature, quality, and success of the work, often set by contract or terms of engagement. Physician writers begin to think of their *emolumentum* as *salarium* rather than *honorarium* and thus must make the case for the nature and dignity of their work and their skills. In doing so, they often argue that the fee is an intrinsic part of the relationship between patient and physician. The patient who knows what care will cost will evaluate it as correspondingly worthwhile and esteem the practitioner as worthy of his earnings. This evaluation will enhance confidence in the physician and so increase the chance for a cure. Only for the poor, who must be treated for the love of God, should the fee be dispensed with, although, as we have seen, doctors like Henri de Mondeville recognized the possibility that the rich could subsidize the poor.[3] The propriety and equity of medical fees in a competitive world of practice becomes a central topic of medical ethics. During the high Middle Ages, St. Thomas Aquinas ironically noted that the power of money had converted the art of healing into the art of moneymaking.[4] Now the question was how to reconcile the two legitimate aims of the profession, healing and income.

Of the three forms of medical ethics—decorum, deontology, and politic ethics—the last has been least apparent so far in the pages of this history. It now begins to grow in prominence. The concern of the state with the practice of medicine begins to show in the Sicilian laws of the early thirteenth century; the concern of practitioners about their place in the state appears as the university-trained physicians seek prominence among the eminent classes of the emerging commercial society of the fourteenth century. A politic ethics seeks to articulate the duties of those whose work is intimately related to the welfare of a political unit, a community. When, in the late medieval period, Italian towns became politically vital and commercially vigorous centers, they provided a milieu that encouraged the growth of a politic ethics. Those towns—Florence, Venice, Bologna, Padua, Vincenza, Verona, Pisa, and many others—valued the work of the new university-trained physicians enough to employ on contract (*condotta*) one or more physicians to care for their populace. Many copies of these contracts have been preserved. They show the city fathers seeking well-trained doctors, inviting them to take up residence and to provide reliable medical service. In some towns, a sort of capitation arrangement was established: the contract doctor was paid a set salary to provide medical service to all citizens. In others, contract doctors agreed to provide free consultation to all citizens and were allowed to charge for treatment. Elsewhere, a fee scale was established whereby the doctor could charge the wealthy but had to serve the poor for free. City doctors also had forensic and public health duties. Strict rules about absence from the city were laid down. These rules became significant when, in 1347, the Black Death, a pandemic of bubonic plague, arrived in Europe and remained endemic for three centuries. Italian town doctors had a legal obligation to stay with the populace, although it is known that they often gave up their position rather than remain; others demanded more money to entice them to risk the danger of death.[5] The Black Death evoked the deontological theme about the obligation of physicians to serve the sick and strenghtened the emerging politic ethics about the role of physicians in the community.

The duty to comfort the sick and dying was a moral imperative common to Christians and Jews, whether they were physicians or not. The bubonic plague, as it swept in successive waves across Europe over the next centuries, thrust that common moral imperative into the consciences of physicians who, while they had no strong tradition of entering danger to care for the sick, recognized that their calling summoned them to greater sacrifice. Although a certain medical optimism is manifested in the multitude of medical treatises about the care and cure of plague victims, each outbreak provoked a crisis of conscience among physicians. Many followed their own advice to their patients, summarized in what was known as the Hippocratic Prescription—*cito, longe, tarde*: "leave fast, go far and return slowly." Plague histories recount many episodes of all or most physicians fleeing a stricken city. At the same time, many physicians remained out of charity, patriotism, or desire for profit.

Theologians spoke out on the duty of doctors to remain with the sick, but their advice was as diverse as their doctrine. Martin Luther, who remained with his flock in the Wittenberg plague of 1527, urged doctors and ministers to fulfill the obligation of Christian charity by faithful service. On the other hand, Theodore Beza, principal disciple of the other great reformer, John Calvin, argued that physicians and ministers could depart if the preservation of their lives was in the interest of the commonwealth. Catholic casuists generally imposed a duty on physicians to remain "in a public peril, such as plague, even at risk of their lives." Rabbinic scholars propounded a duty to flee the plague—the Talmud briskly says, "when plague arrives in town, gather your legs"—only occasionally allowing those who could be useful to the striken community to remain.[6]

Some physicians spoke passionately about their duty to remain with their patients. Guy de Chauliac wrote: "physicians dared not visit the sick for fear of becoming infected. And when they did visit, they did nothing and earned nothing, for all the sick died . . . I, to avoid infamy, did not dare remove myself, but with continuous fear preserved myself as best I could."[7] The father of modern surgery, Ambroise Paré, reflected on the danger of caring for plague victims: "Surgeons must remember that they are called by God to this vocation of surgery, therefore they should go to it with high courage and free of fear, having firm faith that God both gives and takes our lives as and when it pleases Him."[8] Noble sentiments aside, conscientious physicians were caught between the danger of dying and fidelity to the sick. This moral perplexity persisted down to the day when Samuel Pepys listened to the aristocratic Dr. Goddard defend himself and his fellow physicians for leaving plague-ridden London in 1666, "saying that their particular patients were gone out of town."[9] As the pompous Dr. Goddard delivered this apology, a humble apothecary, William Boghurst, stated an ethical ideal. It is said that while the physicians and the Anglican clergy fled, the apothecaries and dissenting ministers, who usually came from, and served, the lower classes, stayed at their posts. Boghurst wrote:

> Everyman that undertakes to bee of a profession or takes on himself an office must take all parts of it, the good and the evill, the pleasure and the pain, the profit and the inconveniences all together and not pick and chuse; for Ministers must preach, Captains must fight and Physitians attend upon the sick.[10]

The ethical debates surrounding the plague moved the politic ethics of medicine ahead: under what circumstances does a person who has medical skills have a special obligation to serve the community?

Another epidemic also drew the work of physicians of that era into close contact with moral beliefs. Syphilis came to Europe in epidemic proportions at the end of the fifteenth century. Named the "French disease," it was quickly recognized as venereal, transmitted in some manner through sexual intercourse. Many medical treatises discussed the origins of the contagion, as well as its modes of transmission, prevention, and treatment. However, the association with sexual intercourse inevitably invited moralizing. Many physician authors repeated the preachers' admonition that this new disease was God's scourge for the sins of a corrupt society and of licentious persons. Some physicians took the moralizing further, urging prevention by total abstention from sex or at least from illicit sex, while refraining from mentioning the widely accepted medical advice about precautions before, during, and after intercourse and the accepted therapeutic drugs, mercury and guaiac. Daniel Sennert, Professor of Medicine at the University of Wittenberg in the early seventeenth century, reproves colleagues who teach medical means of disease prevention, such as the use of condoms or douches: "I do not believe that those things can be taught with a good conscience by which so many men are encouraged to lust, whom perhaps the fear of this disease might have frightened from it."[11] In 1724, the American Puritan preacher Cotton Mather of Boston, who was a medical scholar but not a practitioner, wrote a book of medical advice that was particularly harsh on syphilitic patients. After a tirade against the sin of unchastity, he proclaims: "As for any Remedies under this Foul Disease,—You are so Offensive to me, I'll do nothing for you." Then he relents enough to suggest a course of cathartics that will "keep you in torment for three Days together."[12] Although Mather was a minister rather than a physician, many medical practitioners, firm in their faith, agreed with his severe judgment.

These two epidemics, bubonic plague and syphilis, posed problems on the edge of the emerging world of professional medicine. The question of service to the sick even at the cost of danger to oneself might trouble the conscience of a virtuous person who practiced medicine, but should it be the mark of the profession as a whole? The close link between the medically needed and the morally right might seem appropriate to the believing practitioner, but should a profession break that link and offer treatment, regardless of what the believer might think of the moral dimensions of the disease or the treatment? For the next several centuries, the emerging professions struggled with these questions. Not until the nineteenth century did a general consensus appear, stating that physicians should take personal risks to serve those in need of care and should not render care based upon moral appraisal of the patient's behavior. A latter-day epidemic, AIDS, revived those questions and tested the traditional answers.

It is worthwhile to pause and consider what ethics meant to the educated Renaissance physician. When Jan Yperman, writing in about 1330, recommended that physicians should read books of ethics along with books of physics, he was certainly thinking of Aristotle's *Ethics*, which had been discovered by Western scholars less than a century before and had quickly become the premier text for the academic study of morality. Every university-trained physician would have parsed that text, as well as its companion, *Politics*, and would have found therein the thesis that moral goodness was the achievement of happiness—by the practice of intellectual and moral virtues. Aristotle says little about practical ethical decisions, except to propose that such decisions are made by prudent persons with virtue (although, in saying that, he compares moral with medical decision making).[13] Other books on ethics at that time were commentaries on the complex propositions of Aristotelian doctrine or collections of the maxims of the Christian Fathers. Two centuries later, at the height of the Renaissance, a new authority appeared. Cicero's *De Officiis* (*On Duty*) had been rediscovered and now stood equal or superior to Aristotle. The Roman went beyond descriptions of virtue to a doctrine of natural law wherein one could find, inscribed in the human conscience and condition, precepts that directly guided human behavior. In Cicero's work, politicians, soldiers, lawyers, and merchants could find acute analyses of the problems of telling the truth, keeping promises, and, above all, deciding between personal expedience and the common good. Although medicine was below Cicero's notice, *De Officiis* became a rich source of moral argument about the duties of doctors (his example about whom to save when some shipwrecked persons must be sacrificed reappears in the modern debate about allocation of life support).[14] Thus, the educated physicians of the late Middle Ages and the Renaissance, when advised to study ethics, could turn to the familiar authors of their school days, Aristotle and Cicero. Although few medical writings on ethics allude, in any detail, to these classical authors, they are cited briefly but their doctrines of virtue and duty are always in the background.

During the fifteenth century, Catholic theologians developed a special branch of theology concentrating on the moral duties of Christians. These new moral theologians examined in meticulous detail the duties of various states of life. Medical work was discussed under the heading of the Fifth Commandment of the Decalogue, "Thou shalt not kill," where the moral challenge to physicians who engaged in dangerous work in order to save life was analyzed. In obedience to God, Christians are obliged to protect and preserve their own lives; however, it is unclear how far they must go to fulfill this duty. Theologians developed cases around this question that called for refined analysis (casuistry). One case posed the question: There is an obligation to save one's life; so, must a criminal condemned to burn at the stake pour the cup offered to slake his thirst onto the flames in order to prolong his life for a few seconds? A second, more medical case asked: must a person undergo an excruciating and mutilating surgery to save his or her life? The theologians answered that no one is obliged to preserve life by extraordinary means, which includes any means that would be futile (as in the first case) or require heroic virtue (as in the second case). The language of *ordinary* and *extraordinary* means of preserving life entered the vocabulary of medical morals. When in 1952 Pope Pius XII told a convention of physicians that the newly invented ventilator was an obligatory therapy only if it was an "ordinary means, that is, a means that does not involve any grave burden for oneself or another," he was echoing the teaching of Catholic theologians of the fifteenth century.[15] The same theologians used the theory of *double effect*, first formulated by Thomas Aquinas as a justification of self-defense, to analyze many medical-moral problems: mutilations such as amputation and sterilization, ordinarily forbidden evils, might be justified if their purpose was the saving of life.[16] Around this extensive casuistry a refined medical ethics was elaborated; Catholic doctors and the Catholic faithful were instructed to make decisions about medical care under the guidance of these moral teachings.

The distinguished Italian physician Giovanni Codronchus (1547–1628) applied this moral theology to the work of physicians. In his *Christian and Careful Method of Medicine* (*De Christiana ac Tuta Medendi Ratione*), he discussed many moral problems faced by the practitioner; for example, he wondered whether a physician may accept money for treating an incurable dying person. He concluded that the physician may do so on the condition that he does not conceal the impending death or untruthfully promise a cure. He also warned physicians that they sin if they rejoice that many persons are ill, providing more business. It is particularly wrong to give advice or treatment to healthy persons so that they become ill and thus require the services of the doctor. It is plausible to assume that these curious cases are not entirely figments of Dr. Codronchus' imagination. The physician, concludes Codronchus, may have many virtues, but "if he lack justice, all other virtues will fail him, for justice is the sum and source of all virtues." A Protestant version of this moral theology of medicine is a small book entitled *The Sinning Physician* (*Medicus Peccans*) published in 1684. The author, Ahasverius Fritsch, listed 23 sins commonly committed by physicians, including practicing medicine without sufficient learning, failing to entrust themselves and their patients to divine providence, charging the poor a fee or overcharging the rich, prolonging treatment for the sake of gain, failing to consult when appropriate, abandoning a patient and fleeing the city in contagion, damaging the reputation of other physicians, and revealing the secret vices of patients. Physicians must not prescribe untried medicine or prescribe when drunk. The final sin is to violate the professional oath. Fristch then provided an example of an oath taken by medical graduates of the University of Jena. The graduate vowed to honor the faculty, never to neglect his patients, to charge fees suited to the patient's condition, and never to perform an abortion. He promised not to bring medicine into disrepute and to live an honorable and Christian life.[17]

A new world of medicine had emerged during the late Middle Ages. A medical profession was forming, becoming more commercial and more involved in the affairs of the state. That new world comes into focus in Gabriele de Zerbi's book *Advice to Physicians* (*De Cautelis Medicorum*), published in 1495 in Padua, where he was professor of medicine. This book, called by one historian "the first systematic account of medical ethics,"[18] describes the physician as an educated person of the middle or upper social class whose primary ethical obligation is to earn the trust of patients. The central virtue of the good physician is "fidelity," a notion that is woven through wide-ranging advice about intercourse with patients, fees, and consultations with colleagues. A modern commentator paraphrases Zerbi's theme: "the doctor is the faithful companion of the body of his patient, suffers with him and rejoices in his health. To neglect him, to act improperly in his home, to do anything prohibited by common morality or special medical ethics would be to break faith with the patient."[19] Fidelity extends beyond the patient; the physician must be faithful to the learned tradition of medicine, to other learned and moral colleagues, and to the teaching of the Holy Church, for the rules of morality and of medical ethics rest ultimately on the law of the Gospel. The physician, said Zerbi, is like a priest, to whom God has revealed the divine powers of healing and to whom men reveal their souls for the cure of their bodies. A physician must cultivate a life worthy of such a priesthood. "Zerbi's ethics," says a modern historian, "seem to be one of the earliest expressions of a group's self-regulatory rules of the renaissance period . . . a self-conscious discussion of how medical men should behave."[20] A politic ethics now distinctly joins the classical decorum and the Christian deontology.

Only a quarter of a century after Zerbi's volume was published, physician self-regulation took institutional form in England. In 1511, King Henry VIII complained that "the science and cunning of physick and surgery . . . is daily within this realm exercised by a great multitude of ignorant persons . . . to the grievous hurt, damage and destruction of many of the King's liege people."[21] He ordered that a system of examination and licensure be established under the authority of the Church. Seven years later, a small group of physicians led by the learned Dr. Thomas Linacre, personal physician to Cardinal Wolsey, petitioned the king to charter a College of Physicians with the right to examine all who would practice medicine and to discipline those who violated the rules of the College. Over the next years, the College worked to consolidate its authority over the practice of medicine in the City of London. The College's licensure examination required detailed knowledge of Galen's texts (candidates were required to comment on selected citations that they had to find by memory in the books). Thus, the monopoly of licensed practice went to the socially eminent who enjoyed the privilege of a university education. As one historian writes, "To the College, education in the proper subjects (Latin and Greek classics) and at the proper universities must, above all else, produce a gentleman who was acquainted with the social conventions and preferences of England's ruling class."[22] The proper universities, however, were not enough. On one occasion, the College of Physicians used its broad powers to imprison a certain Dr. Thomas Bonham, who was practicing in London with a degree from Cambridge University. The College claimed that the Cambridge degree in medicine was not a substitute for its own license. Chief Justice Coke wrote an opinion that released Bonham (who later became a lawyer). Coke's opinion was overturned by the King's Bench, leaving the College with extensive control over medical practice.[23] The College issued statutes titled "ethical," virtually all of which dealt with fines and penalties for violation of College rules. These statutes had originally, and correctly, been titled "penal," but Dr. John Caius, College president from 1555 to 1571, added the word "ethical" in 1563 "out of respect for doctoral dignity."[24] By making this change, "Caius's most enduring and dubious accomplishment," says a modern historian, "was the confusion he inflicted in the realm of professional ethics."[25] These statutes are only faintly ethical. Fellows of the College were forbidden to reveal the names of medicines to the common people, "lest they be harmed thereby," and fellows were admonished never to criticize their colleagues in public.[26] Although both rules became deeply embedded in professional ethics, they have been severely criticized in recent times as examples of self-interest masked as ethics. The ethical statutes were "pragmatic devices primarily designed to enhance the status and prosperity of the College itself."[27]

Important treatises on medical ethics appeared in the second half of the sixteenth century and the beginning of the seventeenth.[28] In all these treatises, the decorous physician of Hippocrates, melded with the philosophical physician of Galen, is seen working in an increasingly complex world of scientific and social change. One of these books, Rodrigo à Castro's *Medicus Politicus* (1614), was unique in style and content. À Castro was a Portuguese Jewish physician who spent his medical career in Hamburg. The title page of his volume describes him as "a philosopher and medical doctor celebrated throughout Europe." Credited, like Zerbi's book, as "one of the first modern works on medical ethics," à Castro's book is directed to "physicians, the sick, those who assist the sick and others who cultivate the literary and political disciplines."[29] Although the title, *Medicus Politicus*, recalls Plato's accolade to Asklepios, the author does not cite that classical text. Instead, he applies the phrase to two issues that his book will explain: first, many physicians who claim medical knowledge lack skill in the "political economy" that surrounds medical activities, namely, the manner of conversing with the sick and appreciating their social and economic circumstances; second, medicine is useful to the state only if physicians possess virtue—in particular, the virtues of prudence and generosity—and attain knowledge of medicine based on reason and experience.[30] Medicine suffers disrepute because many *pseudomedici* practice either with no science at all or with the false doctrines of the empiricists, the methodists, and the iatrochemists. À Castro takes great pains to demolish the claims of those sects and also disputes the utility of astrology for medicine. He states that the educated physician must be a master of the humanities, of moral and natural philosophy, and of anatomy and botany. À Castro then describes decorum in the classical fashion: the good physician will be courteous and hospitable to all orders of persons, grave but not morose, familiar but not fatuous, and a devoted husband; he will shun anger, concupiscence, luxury, intemperance, and, above all, "those particularly medical vices . . . almost congenital and hereditary for physicians, avarice, pride and envy."[31]

À Castro adopts a style quite different from that of contemporary books about medical morality. He goes beyond decorum to raise and resolve particular moral problems that the virtuous physician will face. In the manner of the casuistic literature produced by the Catholic moral theologians of his day and the rabbis of his own Jewish tradition, he states each question precisely, defines and distinguishes terms, states the opinions of leading authors from classical philosophy, examines the strength and weakness of arguments on both sides, and proposes a solution. The first of these questions is "whether a physician may deceive the patient for health's sake"—a question "highly controversial." He judges that withholding the truth does not constitute a lie; so, a physician may refrain from full disclosure of the truth, but only if the physician acts with good intent, to help the patient, and not out of avarice. Further, if an untruth is not harmful and is told out of duty (called by the casuists *mendacium officiosum*), a physician may speak deceptively. Still, in principle, a patient "of strong spirit ought to be told the truth, opportunely, gently and without detriment."[32] À Castro performs similar casuistry on a number of other cases: physicians have an obligation to serve all who seek their help, even enemies, although not at the risk of life and limb; they should serve the poor without payment; they should never visit the sick unless invited; and they should care for the ungrateful and should never undertake to cure the incurable.[33]

Friedrich Hoffman, professor of medicine at the University of Halle, also titled his book *Medicus Politicus*. Published in 1749, the book appeared in the midst of the Enlightenment, in the absolutist military state of Prussia. Hoffman's "politic" physician is one who can rationally organize his life, studies and practice in accord with enlightened self-interest. He can circulate at court, with colleagues, and among the sick with confidence ("urbane" might be a better translation than "politic"). The primary medical virtue is prudence, the ability to make rational decisions in complex situations. Hoffman's interpretation of prudence hovers between the Aristotelian-scholastic meaning—the ability to make a virtuous decision in complex circumstances—and the Hobbesian-Enlightenment concept of calculation in promoting one's own interest. The prudent physician will be a Christian (Hoffman himself was a Pietist, a seventeenth-century Protestant sect that stressed the interior spiritual life rather than external ecclesiastical forms of religion), for then "he will necessarily exercise mercy, especially toward the poor, for the merciful God created medicine free and allows it to be practiced out of his goodness."[34] At the same time, the prudent physician will remain decently distant from the poor, lest they become too dependent upon him. "The learned should be dealt with in a learned manner; the ignorant need only be given a general explanation of their affliction."[35] Physicians should not be timid with important persons but should be careful "not to make pretenses of curing the incurable: keep this rule above all when treating princes."[36]

Dr. Hoffman insists on the distinction between physicians and surgeons, based on the rationality and erudition of the former, and also distinguishes the physician from the pharmacist. Detailed advice about intercourse with colleagues and

patients is joined to an extensive discussion of fees. Much of this advice echoes
the traditional decorum but is sensitive to the new structures of education and
society. Hoffman, however, is doing more than giving prudent advice. He is presenting, he believes, an ethic based on the sound philosophical doctrine of Natural Law as expounded by the Dutch jurisprudent Hugo Grotius and by his own
Pietist contemporary at Halle, the philosopher Christian Thomasius. Ethics, in this
view, can be deduced in a logical, almost mathematical, fashion from axioms. Rules
of personal behavior derive from the precepts written by a rational God in a rational nature, capable of being discerned by rational humans. The nature of human
beings gives rise to the nature of medicine, and the nature of medicine gives rise
to the morality of medicine. Dr. Hoffman agrees with Thomasius that "the knowledge of all disciplines, including medical jurisprudence, produces a citizen who
is watchful over the *salus* (meaning both physical health and religious salvation)
of himself and of the body politic."[37] In Hoffman's *Medicus Politicus* the politic
ethics of medicine is more clearly articulated than ever before.

At the close of the eighteenth century, the most elaborate exposition of politic
ethics appeared: Johann Peter Frank's *A System of Complete Medical Police* (1779),
a six-volume treatise on how the state should foster and protect the health of its
people. The title, *Medical Police (Medicinischen Polizey)*, would be translated today
as *Medical Policy* or *Health Policy*. Dr. Frank had served as a country doctor, a
local health officer, chief physician of the Vienna Allgemeines Krankenhaus (then
the world's largest hospital), professor in five universities, and protophysicus of
the Austrian province of Lombardy. His treatise showed how all aspects of the health
of individuals and of the population as a whole, from procreation and parturition
to prostitution, luxurious living, and occupational diseases, from epidemics to
hospital conditions, influenced the general welfare and prosperity of the Austro-
Hungarian Empire. It was the duty of the empire and its rulers to educate people
about health and to create conditions in which they could live safely. Deeply influenced by the political philosophy of Christian Wolff, who envisioned a benignly
paternalistic absolutist state, and even more deeply by Jean Jacques Rousseau's
view that human ills were fomented by the growth of civilization, which crowded
people together in unhealthy cities and lured them away from honest labor, Frank
proposed laws and reforms that would enhance the natural strength and vitality of
the people. In Frank's broad vision, medicine was far more than the care and cure
of individuals; it was "the determination of the rules, based on reason and experience, according to which the creation and multiplication of a strong posterity is
ensured, the present state of health maintained, lost health replaced by a procedure
almost approaching creation, and death and decay relegated to the outermost boundaries of an attainable age." His view of the role of the physician is striking:

> Philanthropic physicians should investigate the nature, situation and condition of
> the smallest village, its diseases and their causes, the ratio of its sexes, of the differ-
> ent classes of men, calculate the ratio of births and deaths, and thus produce a kind

of geography of each district. This geography would indicate the boundaries of life and death, the width and length of the dangerous lakes, and the safest routes between the reefs on which many thousands founder because of mere ignorance. The saving of individual persons must be viewed as a greater deed than the conquering of a province.

This "geography," which today would be called epidemiology, guides the physician in correcting social conditions as he heals individuals. The civic duties of physicians and the profession are incorporated in this vision. Frank anticipated the science of social medicine and the functions of public health, and his thesis that public health contributed to public prosperity inspired even Bismark's support of state health insurance. However, that thesis could also cultivate a view of medicine and its practitioners at the service of the state. Frank indignantly denied that his medical police "outrageously limits innate personal rights, which have already been curtailed too much; violates the rights of fathers, husbands, and parents, and . . . gives these into the hands of a despotic government."[38] Yet, a century after his death, his benign paternalism was distorted by the Nazi state into *racial hygiene*, the servile, statist medicine that discarded those who could not meet the standards of Aryan fitness.[39] Despite this hideous misinterpretation, Frank's thinking expanded the politic ethics of medicine beyond the reciprocal exchange of public service for professional prestige. The medical profession on the European continent developed within a much stronger culture of state control of medicine than did the British and American professions, and duties to the common good of populations were as much a part of their ethics as duties to individual patients.

By the end of the eighteenth century, politic ethics had come into its own. The practice of medicine everywhere was the work of a profession. Although many persons of diverse training and talents offered medical services of all sorts outside the professional sphere, a corps of educated practitioners gradually achieved social and economic prominence sufficient to claim the right to restrict medical practice to their own kind. In some places, these prominent professionals, organized into colleges with memberships of their own choosing, were granted the right to license; in others, the state controlled licensure but under the powerful influence of the profession. In order to demonstrate their utility to the commonwealth and to develop trust among potential patients, physicians had to appear useful and trustworthy. Thus, an ethic of competence and compassion was politic, that is, expedient for the success of the profession. At the same time, the profession undertook certain responsibilities for the common welfare, and many of its practitioners, who benefited from the politic ethics, internalized its principles, accepting as their own the values of competence and compassion within the wider moral compass of public service. Thus, the politic ethics of the profession is intrinsically ambiguous: it can refer either to the expedient, self-serving adaptation of the profession to public expectations or to the internalized morality of practitioners who really believe that, as physicians, they are held to a high standard of public accountability for their professional behavior. To the traditional decorum and deontology are added a few public responsibilities but, more important, the entire set of ethical requisites is raised to a higher power of public responsibility.

The emergence of a profession and of its attendant politic ethics fosters a new style of expressing medical ethics in the form of a code. Roman law had been published in *Codices*, collections of imperial and legal rulings. During the eighteenth century, European jurisprudence was captivated by the succinct, organized structure of the Roman codes, and scholars attempted to encapsulate the untidy legal instruments of a long, complex history into modern equivalents. The Napoleonic reform of French law was the great achievement of this effort. A similar effort to compose tidy proclamations of the medical profession's beliefs about its own probity and dedication to the public began to appear. In postrevolutionary France, groups of all sorts devised codes of honor, "guides to comportment that . . . taught men how they must act to earn worldly renown, avoid conflict with each other and prosper with each other in accord with a standard of egalitarian chivalry." French medical society followed suit, portraying the medical man as "*un parfait honnête homme*, moved by loyalty and courtesy to fellows and patients."[40] The first explicit medical code appeared in the same era, Thomas Percival's *Medical Ethics; or, a Code of Institutes and Precepts Adapted to the Professional Conduct of Physicians and Surgeons* (1803). This book, destined to become highly influential in the English-speaking world, will be fully discussed in the following chapter.

The actual influence of the high-minded literature about medical deontology and decorum on the lives and practices of physicians is difficult to ascertain. In classical times, popular literature depicts physicians as greedy, ignorant rascals. They receive no better treatment from the secular authors of the era of scholarly medicine. Chaucer's "verry parfit praktisour" of Physik is praised as learned in "Olde Ypocras, Haly and Galyen, Razis and Avycen," but "he kepte the gold he wan in pestilence, for gold in physik is a cordial, therefore he lovede gold in special" (cynical as it is, this text does tell us that the doctor treated plague patients). The three literary greats of France—François Rabelais, Michel de Montaigne, and Molière—ridiculed the scholarly pretensions of medical men. Rabelais, a physician himself, depicts a certain Dr. Rondibilis as a garrulous pedant, spouting Hippocratic texts and proudly prescribing remedies recommended "by a celebrated author dead eighteen hundred years." Montaigne's essay "On the Resemblance of Children to Their Fathers" may be the most devastating attack on doctors ever written. He writes, "as far as my knowledge goes, I see no group of people so soon sick and so late cured as those who are under the jurisdiction of medicine." This is so, claims Montaigne, "because the most important science . . . being the one that is in charge of our preservation and health, is unfortunately the most uncertain, the most confused, and agitated by the most changes." In Molière's

Malade imaginaire, Argan, the hypochondriac, is induced into the profession, *in nostro docto corpore*, by passing a ridiculous examination administered by pompous doctors. In his less well known *L'Amour médecin*, four doctors argue over the best remedy for the patient, who eventually recovers without their help, much to their anger. "It is better to die according to the rules," says Dr. Bahys, "than to recover contrary to them." In the rarely performed *Monsieur de Pourceaugnac*, Molière depicts a physician seeking a patient who has escaped from his unwanted care; the offended doctor proclaims, "his disease, which I have been told to cure, is my property. . . . he has been placed under my care and he is obliged to be my patient. . . . I shall have him condemned by decree to be cured by me."[41] The playwright himself answered King Louis XIV, who had asked him how he got along with his own doctor: "Sire, we talk. He prescribes remedies. I do not take them and I recover."[42] Satires against doctors in this era attacked not only traditional medical greed but also the prized scholarship of the emerging profession.

Again, we cannot know how pervasive among practitioners were the faults ridiculed by the satirists. An English physician traveling in Italy in 1600 commented favorably on the university-trained physicians of that country, in obvious contrast with his own British colleagues:

> The Universities of Siena and Salernum of old and espetailly of Padoa as well of old as of this day have yielded famous phisitians who in Italy are also shirgians and many of them growe rich for all that have any small means will in sicknes have their helpe, because they are not prowde but will looke upon any ordure and handle any sore, but espetially because they are carefull for their patients, visite them diligently and take little fees which make heavy purses. They visite twise each day the poorest patient.[43]

At the end of the era surveyed in this chapter, a physician's face peers out from a portrait that, in visage at least, manifests the virtues of the profession. One of Goya's most poignant etchings shows his very sick self being tenderly embraced by an obviously concerned and compassionate "Dr. Arrieta, his physician." How many Dr. Arrietas moved among the pretentious grandees of medicine?

5

British Medicine
Eighteenth and Nineteenth Centuries

In eighteenth-century England, medicine was a learned and gentlemanly profession. The ethics of that profession was framed by courtesy, the behavior proper to gentlemen, taught in a torrent of popular literature on social manners that had begun with Thomas Elyot's *Book Named the Governor* (1531). This literature combined advice about etiquette with reflections on moral virtue; some volumes reflected ethical sincerity and others, like Lord Chesterfield's *Letters to His Son* (1774), profound cynicism. Sincere or cynical, the writings presented the gentleman as the paragon of morality and gentlemanliness as the prime virtue. This literature provided the model for medical ethics in seventeenth- and eighteenth-century England.[1] Standards of aristocratic behavior, marked pervasively by respect for status, governed the physician and all his social equals. However, gentlemanliness did not banish an intense competition among practitioners for prestige and patients. British physicians found it difficult to develop lucrative practices and often denigrated the competence and character of rivals. The Royal Colleges were engaged in constant disputes with practitioners who did not hold their license and in frequent quarrels with their own members. The political, class, and religious differences of early Hanoverian England aggravated the medical disputes.[2]

At the same time, a more benign impulse stimulated the founding of voluntary hospitals, or infirmaries, in many British towns. Groups of prominent persons, often with distinguished physicians among them, aimed "to infuse a Christian and charitable spirit into the operation of the Poor Law," which "lay harshly on the impoverished sick."[3] The wealthy founders of the infirmaries were entitled to admit persons of their choice for medical and nursing treatment and supervision. Seventeen of these infirmaries appeared in England between 1718 and 1750. Since the founders and governors engaged the physicians and surgeons, disputes were bound to arise over the choice of persons who were professionally, religiously, and politically suitable to serve on the medical and surgical staffs. George Eliot's

1871 novel *Middlemarch*,[4] set in an English provincial town in the early nineteenth century, vividly portrays a fictional dispute of that sort.

An actual dispute rent the staff and governors of the Manchester Infirmary at the end of the eighteenth century. Hospital posts had been divided between Tory surgeons and Dissenting and Whig physicians, to no one's satisfaction.[5] In 1791, the governors of the Manchester Infirmary invited Dr. Thomas Percival, a leading physician of the city, to prepare a "scheme of professional conduct relative to hospitals and other medical charities." Dr. Percival, who had studied medicine first at Edinburgh and had graduated from the University of Leyden, was a man of high culture and philosophical interests, as well as a leader in public health and hospital regulation. His essay, finished a year later, circulated privately for comment among many of his friends and was finally published in 1803 as *Medical Ethics; or, a Code of Institutes and Precepts, Adapted to the Professional Conduct of Physicians and Surgeons*.[6] This title is the debut of the term *medical ethics* in the literature of medical morality. Percival chose it after some commentators objected to the provisional title, *Medical Jurisprudence*. He explained that he saw jurisprudence and ethics as similar, citing Justinian's definition of jurisprudence: *juris praecepta sunt haec: honeste vivere, alterum non laedere, suum cuique tribuere* (the precepts of law are: live morally, hurt no one, give to each his due).[7] Percival might also have been thinking of Justinian when he designated his work as a code, for the emperor's laws had been collected in a *Codex* in which each law is stated in a short paragraph. Percival remarked that he had written "in an aphoristic form . . . [which] forbids all digression."[8] This code style, and the name itself, would be a model for statements of professional ethics in the future.

Percival set out "to frame a general system of medical ethics; that the official conduct, and mutual intercourse of the faculty, might be regulated by precise and acknowledged principles of urbanity and rectitude."[9] *Medical Ethics* is divided into four chapters: on duties relative to hospitals, professional conduct in private practice, relations with apothecaries, and duties relative to the law. Underlying all duties was the moral notion that the physician should be a "gentleman" in all his dealings with patients and with colleagues. In the Dedication, written to his son, a medical student, Percival writes, "the study of professional ethics . . . will soften your manners, expand your affections, and form you to that propriety and dignity of conduct, which are essential to the character of a gentleman."[10] *Gentleman*, in the moral parlance of the time, signified not only an array of decorous, amiable behaviors but also certain fundamental virtues. The gentleman physician "must unite tenderness with steadiness, and condescension with authority, as to inspire the minds of their patients with gratitude, respect and confidence."[11] Consistent attention to the care of the patient marks Percival's advice, urging that attending physicians advocate the welfare of the patient against the parsimony of the governors, who are always inclined to overcrowd and to use cheap medicines. Hospital patients, the sick poor, should be provided the same care as private patients. Percival insists that disputes about the competence of practitioners or about the care of patients should be settled by collective judgment of the professional staff. In these ways, Percival created an ethic for a new medical milieu, the eighteenth-century hospital, in which multiple practitioners shared the care of patients who were generally needy and of a social class distinctly below that of their patrons and physicians. The virtue of "condescension" that he urges does not mean supercilious patronizing, but rather the acceptance of one's social inferior as an equal.

Percival's sonorous prose rolls through some 72 precepts in the first three chapters, counseling sympathy and patience with patients, sensitivity in communication and confidentiality, courtesy, firm discretion, and respect for precedence in dealing with colleagues and consultants. The fourth chapter, which concerns duties relative to the law, is a treatise on medical jurisprudence, informing physicians about their roles as witnesses in criminal cases and as guardians of the public health. Percival's *Medical Ethics* repeats much of the classical decorum, expressed in the language of a Georgian-era English gentleman, but it also moves this decorum into the new world of complex social relationships between professionals with differing competencies working together in an institution within an urban industrial society. In Percival's view, the physician had acquired the duties of "office," granted to them by society: "Let the physician and surgeon never forget that their professions are public trusts. . . ."[12] Percival explicitly borrowed this notion from a friend, the moralist Thomas Gisborne. Reverend Gisborne was the author of the widely praised *Enquiry into the Duties of Men*, which Percival called, "the most complete system extant of Practical Ethics."[13] Both Gisborne and Percival saw the office of physician, with its attendant duties, within the larger framework of the duties of individuals to the society. Percival's *Medical Ethics*, so thoroughly permeated with the classical decorum, was at the same time an expression of the politic ethics of medicine.

Gisborne's *Enquiry* contained a section on the moral duties of physicians that Percival appreciated. On one point, Dr. Percival disagrees with his moralist friend. In "Notes and Illustrations," appended to the text of *Medical Ethics*, Percival discusses the delicate matter of telling the truth to patients. He notes that Dr. Samuel Johnson had complained about physicians who "tell lies to the sick man for fear of alarming him. 'You have no business with consequences,' says he, 'you are to tell the truth. . . . Of all lying, I have the greatest abhorrence of this, because I believe it has been frequently practiced on myself'."[14] The complaint of that prestigious patient does not impress Dr. Percival. Reverend Gisborne's defense of truth-telling, which would have pleased Dr. Johnson, is subjected to courteous criticism. The reverend moralist had argued that the physician is "invariably bound never to represent the uncertainty or danger as less than he actually believes it to be, and whenever he conveys, directly or indirectly, to the patient or to his family, any impression to that effect, though he may be misled by mistaken tenderness, he is guilty of positive falsehood." Percival, an experienced physician, begs to differ with the moralist. Drawing on arguments of the moral philosopher Francis Hutcheson, he maintains that if "men do not conceive it an injury to be deceived, there is no crime in false speech about such matters." He writes a succinct essay to support his claim that beneficent deception, which "can lift the drooping spirits" of the sick, is ethical. In special situations, it would be "a gross and unfeeling wrong to reveal the truth" when the truthful answer might prove fatal to the inquirer: "His right to the truth is suspended, and even annihilated; because its beneficial nature being reversed, it would be deeply injurious to himself, to his family and to the public." The patient can be deceived without tainting the "delicate sense of veracity," which the physician must ever honor, for his motive is to benefit, not injure. Percival's essay on truth-telling is a rare instance of sustained philosophical argument on an ethical problem in medical practice. He invites "medical readers [who] wish to investigate this nice and important subject of casuistry" to consult the works of Hugo Grotius, Samuel Pufendorf, Joseph Butler, Francis Hutcheson, and William Paley. His argument convinced many physicians, and, as the next chapter will show, it stood almost unchallenged until the American physicians, Worthington Hooker and Richard Cabot, attacked it.[15]

Percival also appreciated "the excellent lectures of Dr. Gregory." *Lectures Upon the Duties and Qualifications of a Physician* had been published in 1772 by Dr. John Gregory, professor of physic at the University of Edinburgh. Gregory practiced medicine in the flourishing philosophical world of Scotland, where Francis Hutcheson, David Hume, Adam Smith, Thomas Reid, and others were making major contributions to moral philosophy. His lectures address the "genius, understanding and temperament" that suit a man to be a physician, the physician's moral qualities, such as humanity, honor, patience, attendance, discretion, and the "decorum . . . the general propriety of manners and behavior toward patients and fellow physicians, surgeons and apothecaries." In all these topics, Gregory reiterates the themes of the classical decorum literature (he recognizes the ambiguity of the term *decorum*, distinguishing manners founded in nature and common sense from those founded in caprice and fashion).[16]

Gregory attempts to ground his view of the moral qualities proper to physicians on a sound philosophical foundation. He quite naturally borrows the notions popular in the philosophical circle in which he moved. In particular, he adapts the basic concept of his friend and Edinburgh colleague, David Hume: the entire moral life is founded on a natural and intuitive sympathy with the moral sentiments of others. The central duty of the physician, deriving from sympathy, is to relieve suffering and cure disease; from this duty, all other duties, such as confidentiality, flow. Gregory writes, "The chief of these [moral qualities required of a physician] is humanity; that sensibility that makes us feel for the distresses of our fellow-creatures, and which, of consequence, incites us in the most powerful manner to relieve them. Sympathy produces an anxious attention to a thousand little circumstances that may tend to relieve the patient; an attention which money can never purchase: hence the inexpressible comfort of having a friend for a physician."[17] It is this moral basis that distinguishes physicians who are dedicated to the art of medicine from those who use it as a mere article of trade to make a living. Gregory maintains that only the moral physician, guided by sympathy, can benefit patients, for it is by sympathy that the physician engages the affections of the patient, enhancing the probability of an effective cure. Other practitioners of medicine, motivated by gain, merely carry on what he and others disdainfully call "the sick trade."

Gregory's *Lectures* argue that physicians must preserve confidentiality, attend to the wishes of their patients about their treatment (an idea rarely expressed in the literature of medical ethics), tell the truth to patients when their situation is perilous, stay with the dying and the hopelessly ill, and dress and bear themselves in decent and gentlemanly fashion. Historians are beginning to see Gregory's attempt to apply a distinct theory of morality to the practice of medicine as "a fundamental reconceptualization of medical morality." He should stand, they believe, as Percival's equal, or even superior in some respects, as an "inventor" of modern medical ethics.[18]

The serious efforts of physicians such as Gregory and Percival to improve the manners and morals of the profession attest to the sorry state of the profession in their days. Hogarth's cartoons depict clatches of pompous, arrogant, quarrelsome physicians (brought to screen life in the film *The Madness of King George*). Yet physicians of a different sort can be glimpsed in the literature of the time. Samuel Johnson, no great friend of physicians, had a deep affection for a poorly trained, peculiar "practitioner of physik" named Robert Levit. Johnson's elegy for Levit described him as

> Officious, innocent, sincere,
> Of every friendless name the friend . . .
> Obscurely wise, and coarsely kind . . .
> When fainting nature called for aid,
> And hovering death prepared the blow,
> His vigorous remedy displayed
> The power of art without the show . . .
> No summons mocked by chill delay,
> No petty gain disdained by pride,
> The modest wants of every day
> The toil of every day supplied.[19]

A generation later, *Middlemarch*'s Dr. Lydgate, high-minded and highly trained (London, Paris, and Edinburgh), was convinced that despite the ignorance, arrogance, and pettiness of his colleagues, "the medical profession as it might be was the finest in the world; presenting the most perfect interchange between science and art; offering the most direct alliance between intellectual conquest and social good. . . . He cared not only for 'cases' but for John and Elizabeth."[20] There may have been many Levits and Lydgates, who welcomed the words of men such as Gregory and Percival, hearing them not as condemnations but as invitations to generous service.

After these significant works at the end of the eighteenth century and the beginning of the nineteenth, Great Britain produced little original work in medical ethics for more than a century. The debates over medicine's place in society, which stimulated American medical ethics in the nineteenth century, did not take place in England, where the medical profession was regulated and organized earlier and more effectively than in the United States. A legal system for reporting and disciplining those charged with unprofessional conduct was established by the mid-nineteenth century. Physicians, sensitive to their public respectability, endeavored to be above scandal. While ethical disputes did arise, particularly over gynecological surgery and confinement of persons with mental and infectious diseases (both were deemed excessive and often unnecessary), these disputes were generally handled within the profession itself.[21] As the British medical historian Roy Porter writes, "In a characteristically British manner, professional bodies judged that the decision must be left to the doctor's scruples. The ingrained habits of individuality, specific to English liberal politics, and the cult of the gentleman that formed the unspoken code of male elites . . . meant that in professional eyes and, to a large degree, equally in the public mind the ethical dilemmas raised by medicine were best handled not by the law courts, jurists, academic philosophers or Parliament but by the integrity of private practitioners following clinical judgment and their own consciences."[22] Percival's work was never as popular in his homeland as it was in the United States. Codes of ethics did not proliferate among British practitioners, as they did among Americans. We shall now "cross the pond" to watch the long tradition of medical ethics become American.

6

Ethics in American Medicine

British medicine came to North America with the early colonists, who brought its pharmacopoeia but little of its learning. American doctors in the eighteenth century were mostly self-taught or apprenticeship-trained. Any doctor could take on apprentices, and no system, either of regulation or education, imposed any pattern. A few books on the doctor's shelf, most of them of ancient vintage, provided the only references for theory and practice. The rough, haphazard medical world of the early colonies distressed those Americans who were familiar with the more sophisticated and learned world of British medicine. A small stream of Americans went abroad to study in Edinburgh, London, Paris, and other European centers and returned with a yearning to bring scholarly medicine to the colonies. Still, on the eve of the American Revolution, among some 3500 colonial practitioners, only 350 had degrees from European medical schools. Efforts to elevate and educate the profession began with the founding of medical colleges at Philadelphia (1765), King's College of New York (1768), Harvard College (1783), and Dartmouth College (1798). By 1800, ten medical colleges existed in the United States. Immigrant physicians also arrived from many places in Europe, among them a number of well-educated Pietists from the University of Halle who came to serve the German populations of Pennsylvania and South Carolina.[1]

An ethical debate occurred at the very beginning of scholarly medicine in America. The debate had begun in England. In 1714, informants of the Royal College of Physicians had reported a Middle Eastern practice in which dried pus from a smallpox victim was transferred to an unaffected person. This *inoculated* person experienced a brief episode of illness and was afterward protected from the full disease. The Royal College of Physicians, urged by Lady Mary Montagu, wife of the British ambassador to Turkey, was determined to promote the practice. Many practitioners strenuously resisted, protesting that it was unethical to give someone a disease. A series of experiments during the 1720s showed that inoculation, while it did induce disease, prevented more serious disease and death, and the medical profession was slowly converted. The British government had cooper-

63

ated in the experiments, and medicine had found one of its first effective preventive health measures.[2]

The fight to introduce inoculation into America involved a strange cast of characters. Smallpox was a scourge of the colonies. A leading Boston clergyman, Cotton Mather, was deeply interested in medicine. He had authored a book, *The Angel of Bethesda*, that was a curious mixture of theological homily and medical information.[3] In 1715, Mather's Negro servant had told him that in Africa smallpox was prevented by transferring pus from infected persons to healthy ones. Soon thereafter, Mather read the report about Turkish inoculation that had been published in the *Transactions of the Royal Society*. When smallpox next struck Boston, Mather encouraged the town's physicians to inoculate its citizens. All physicians but one, Dr. Zabdiel Boylston, refused. The town's physicians then protested loudly and attempted to force the civic authorities to prevent further inoculation. James and Benjamin Franklin's *New England Courant* fomented the protest, and the public sided with the physicians and the press.

The Boston clergy, including Mather's father, Increase Mather, retired president of Harvard College, supported their colleague and Dr. Boylston. The reluctant doctors had stepped incautiously on theological grounds, claiming that inoculation was not only dangerous but also impious, presuming to deny God's providence in sending the disease. The pastors issued an eloquent refutation of that theological claim, noting that all medicine could be subject to the same indictment. In the end, Dr. Boylston's inoculated patients had an extraordinarily low rate of infection: 2 percent in contrast to the 15 percent in the general population. Reverend Mather reported this success to the Royal Society. He explained the efficacy of inoculation by a theory of animalcular transmission of disease, which presaged later theories of microbial infection. Over the next decades the practice of inoculation came into medical favor, although not until Dr. Edward Jenner introduced the much less dangerous practice of vaccination in 1798 did this early form of immunological prophylaxis win almost universal support. It is intriguing to see this first American debate over medical ethics: theologians advance scientific claims to support a medical innovation against doctors who appropriate theological arguments to defend their conservatism.

As scholarly medicine took hold in the colonies, the small cadre of learned practitioners began to form medical societies to encourage medical study and to improve the ethics of physicians. Physicians in New Jersey organized a Medical Society in 1766 and immediately promulgated a code of ethics, urging medical practitioners to attain learning and to consult only with learned colleagues. In 1769 the first graduating class from King's College heard their professor, Samuel Bard, deliver "A Discourse on the Duties of a Physician." Dr. Bard commences by congratulating the young men who are entering "a profession hitherto (at least in a regular manner) uncultivated among us . . . in the practice of which Integrity and Abilities will place you among the most useful; and Ignorance and Dishonesty among the most pernicious members of society." Bard repeats much of the classical decorum but bases it, as John Gregory would a few years later, on Scottish moral philosophy. The ethics of a physician derive from the "springs of morality," duty and benevolence, as taught by the Scottish philosopher Francis Hutcheson. The virtuous physician is obliged to serve the needs of others even if they cannot compensate him for his services. There is no excuse for errors of ignorance. Finally, Dr. Bard exhorted the graduates, "I would recommend you seriously to consider the Sixth Commandment, 'Thou Shalt Do No Murder'."[4]

Dr. Benjamin Rush of Philadelphia was America's preeminent physician at the time of the Revolution.[5] A signer of the Declaration of Independence, he exhibited an exuberant medical patriotism: America was the healthiest environment (especially "the enlightened and happy state of Connecticut"), not only because of the physical environment but also because republican liberty fostered physical health. America (particularly the province of Pennsylvania) was where "the sciences, ever fond of the company of liberty and industry, chose this spot for the seat of their empire." America's "untrodden fields and forests" would enlarge the *materia medica*, providing "antidotes to those diseases which are supposed to be incurable."[6] Dr. Rush had a broad interest in moral issues. His *Essays Literary, Moral and Philosophical* contained chapters on liberal education, education of women (he supported both), the death penalty, Negro slavery, and the use of tobacco (he opposed all three).

Dr. Rush's lectures to the University of Pennsylvania medical students on "The Institutes and Practice of Medicine" always included ample treatment of morality in medicine. One lecture, "On the Virtues and Vices of Physicians," epitomizes the decorum tradition: the good physician has the virtues of piety and humanity. Humanity implies self-sacrifice, sympathy, service and contribution to the poor, candor and generosity, and, reflecting Dr. Rush's love of country, patriotism and devotion to peace and liberty. Physicians must avoid the vices of impiety, undue confidence in the human power of healing, drunkenness, falsehood and deception, avarice, and obstinacy.[7] Even his lecture "On the Means of Acquiring Business in the Profession of Medicine" is a moralistic treatise: the young physician will develop a successful and profitable practice by application to study, punctuality in visiting the sick, assiduous attendance to the poor, and sympathy with the sick; those physicians who curry favor, cultivate the wealthy, employ faddish remedies, and have offensive manners will never succeed.[8]

The students were treated to "The Duties of a Physician and the Methods of Improving Medicine" as the finale of the course. After extolling the virtues of farm living for country practitioners (rural living was healthier, an ample herb garden could be cultivated, and the poultry and seed that were the doctor's frequent fee could be kept), Rush urged on them the usual decorum of doctors. They should avoid singularity and extravagance in manners, attend divine services regularly, and show themselves to be composed, punctual, and reasonable. "Yield to [patients]," he advised, "in matters of little consequence, but maintain an inflexible authority over them in matters that are essential to life." The physician must be temperate in the use of ardent spirits, especially where the hospitality of families offers "a draught of strong liquor every time he enters into the house of a patient." He should "inspire as much hope of a recovery as [he] can, consistent with truth." Physicians should not abandon patients whose condition seems desperate, for "it is impossible to tell in such cases where life ends and death begins." Advice about charging for services is given, with the special admonition that, "the poor . . . should be the objects of your particular care. Dr. Boerhaave [a Dutch physician of the first half of the seventeenth century] used to say, 'they were his best patients, because God was their paymaster'. . . . [W]henever you are called to visit a poor patient, imagine you hear the voice of the good Samaritan sounding in your ears, 'Take care of him, and I will repay thee'." This lecture remains largely in the decorum tradition, but Dr. Rush phrases the decorum in terms of deontological imperatives: "In visits to the sick, never appear to be in a hurry"; "Avoid making light of any case"; "Do not condemn or oppose unnecessarily the simple prescriptions of your patients"; "Preserve, upon all occasions, a composed or cheerful countenance"; "Never be angry at anything a sick man says or does to you"; "Avoid giving a patient over in acute diseases." These short imperatives, each marked with a Roman numeral like the commandments of the Decalogue, give these counsels the look of a code.[9]

One lecture, "On the Duty of Patients to their Physician," seems an odd one to deliver to medical students. Rush explains that he gives it so that the young practitioners will know how to educate their patients in their duties. First among these is the duty to select a physician with a proper medical education and good personal and moral habits. Physicians should instruct their patients to be candid in discussing their medical problems, to be "prompt, strict and universal" in complying with the doctor's prescriptions, to be considerate of the physician's heavy schedule, and to pay the physician for services, when possible. This last duty is accompanied by a long justification of fair remuneration based on physicians' dedication to their patients, their rigorous education, and their willingness to expose themselves to danger as they cared for the sick. Rush advises his students that "performance of these duties by patients is inseparably connected not only with our rights and interests but with the success of our practices and the advancement of our science." From the perspective of moral philosophy, this lecture is more a deontology than a decorum. The concept of the reciprocity of rights and duties, a common philosophical doctrine, is briefly mentioned but not developed. Among all of Benjamin Rush's words about medical ethics, this particular lecture is destined to survive, as this chapter will soon relate.[10]

The medical faculties of Pennsylvania, Columbia, Harvard, Yale and Dartmouth desired to bring to America the scholarly medicine of Edinburgh, London, and Paris. Educated physicians felt that the profession's standing in society depended not only on scholarship but also on its reputation for ethical behavior. In 1809, the Association of Boston Physicians issued the "Boston Medical Police" (*police*, as in Johann Frank's treatise, was a commonly used word for policy or regulation), based upon the writings of Gregory, Percival, and Rush. That short document stated principles for consultation among practitioners and fees (reinforcing the ancient duty to care for the poor without payment by citing Dr. Rush's quotation of Dr. Boerhaave's remark that God was the paymaster of the poor).[11] In 1819, Dr. Samuel Brown of the Transylvania Medical School in Lexington, Kentucky, founded the Kappa Lambda Society of Aesculapius, a secret society whose members swore to abide by Percival's code. Kappa Lambda promised to become a strong force for medical reform but, ironically, became a center for the promotion of its members' self-interest; its reputation turned "notorious," and it broke up within a few years.[12] Other medical societies devised codes of ethics, often incorporating Percival's language but stressing in notable detail the etiquette of consultation. These included the medical societies of New Hampshire (1819), the District of Columbia (1820), New York (1823), and Maryland (1832).

Codes of ethics were weak remedies for the disdain in which the American public held the profession. Many practitioners were hardly educated, barely literate, dirty, and dangerous. The more educated and competent practitioners were often quarrelsome and contentious among themselves. Medical students had the reputation of being unruly and coarse. One major newspaper referred to the profession as a "stupendous humbug," and a medical paper stated, "it is fashionable to speak of the Medical Profession as a body of jealous, quarrelsome men, whose chief delight is the annoyance and ridicule of each other." In 1838, the New Orleans Physico-Medical Society expelled a certain Dr. Luzenberg with the public denunciation that he was "abrupt in speech, uncouth in manners, irritable and petulant in temper, and arrogant and overbearing in his demeanor." In addition to these breaches of decorum, Dr. Luzenberg used the corpses of patients who had died under his care for target practice! Dr. Luzenberg may have been particularly egregious, but there were enough bad doctors in the first half of the nineteenth century to tarnish the reputation of the entire profession.[13]

Still, among the rascals and ignoramuses there were good doctors. A casebook written by Rev. Charles Devol, M.D., who apparently practiced in upstate New York in the 1840s, reveals the sentiments of a good doctor of that era. After many pages reporting diagnoses and treatment of his patients (for "costiveness, weakness and want of appetite, mix 3 drams magnesium sulfate into one quart of gin, take a tablespoonful 2 or 3 times a day or *pro re nata*"), Devol writes an essay, presumably for his eyes only, on "The Relations of the Physician." "The pure and noble sentiment [to relieve a sufferer] must always prevail, to make the practice of medicine answer its ideal, and render it a blessing to both physician and patient. To live for others and not for himself is a physician's vocation . . . always ready to sacrifice his repose, advantages and comforts, yea even higher considerations, to the end of saving the life and health of his fellow men." The duties of careful attention to the sick and free care for the poor are extolled; the absolute obligation to refrain from "shortening the days of a man, even one who prays for death as an end to his sufferings," is emphasized. Even unproven treatments must be applied to those fatal conditions in which all else has failed, even though failure may tarnish his reputation, for it is not "hope of success but an honest intention which is to direct his actions." Reverend Dr. Devol concludes his essay with a declaration that has the tone of a prayer: "I am not regardless either of wealth or fame [but] may never the desire of either be the moving spring of my actions. . . . May I watch over my patients with all the sollicitude of a father, to attend upon them my sweetest labour, to save them my dearest happiness." We know very little about this pastoral practitioner: his book contains no hint of where or how he was educated, few quotations from the medical authorities, and no clues about his relations with other medical men. If he acted in accord with his sentiments, he must have been a comforting friend in illness (and the epsom salts in gin may have helped) and a notable contrast to the practitioners so reviled by the public.[14]

At about the time Dr. Devol was prescribing his orthodox remedies, another medical influence was infiltrating the new nation. During the third and fourth decades of the nineteenth century, the homeopathic doctrines of Samuel Hahnemann entered the United States with German families who settled first in Pennsylvania and then in New York and Massachusetts. In 1835, Drs. Henry Detwiller and Constantine Herring founded the North American Academy of Homeopathic Healing in Allentown, Pennsylvania. Many physicians and many of the public were attracted to homeopathy, among them Henry Wadsworth Longfellow, Nathaniel Hawthorne, Louisa May Alcott, and Daniel Webster. The system, which in essence claimed that diseases were cured by administration of infinitesimal doses of drugs that caused symptoms similar to the disease, not only brought relief from the heroic and horrific treatments of orthodox physicians but also had a spiritual aura about it. As one historian writes, "Another reason for Hahnemann's popularity stemmed from the troubled spirit of the American romantics during the decades preceding the Civil War. The burgeoning prosperity of the new nation, the travails of industrialism, and the awakened response to new individualism and the uneasy religious conscience, a relic of the Puritan past, left their mark upon a generation of intellectuals seeking new sources of truth and righteousness."[15] Homeopathy relied more on spiritual forces and the recuperative powers of nature than on the minimalist drugs it used.

Many other types of medicine, such as Samuel Thompson's botanical healing, Vincent Priessnitz's hydropathy, and eclectic medicine, appeared in the decades before the Civil War. By 1847 there were 80 medical schools in the United States, but many of them were under the aegis of medical sectarians. At the same time, faith healing burst into popularity in religious circles. Although all states had a legal system of medical licensure at the beginning of the nineteenth century, one by one, starting with Illinois in 1826, state legislatures repealed their licensure laws until, by the time of the Civil War, no effective medical licensure existed in any state. The popular egalitarian spirit of the Jacksonian era fueled the repeal movement. It was asserted that licensure was legislation favoring a single class and that, after all, no sound evidence could distinguish between the different medical sects. Speaking of Jacksonian antielitism, one author says, "In attacking the bugbear of elitism, Jacksonian society cast its vote for no standards at all."[16]

In the midst of this confusion, a desire for order began to be felt. Some of the more educated physicians sincerely desired to restore not only order but also respect for a profession that was widely vilified. Many leaders of the profession felt that improved medical education was the essential antidote to the disrepute into which they judged medicine had fallen. One of these, young Dr. Nathan Smith Davis, proposed to the New York Medical Society resolutions recommending a standard curriculum and state licensure independent of medical school degree. His resolutions were not only adopted but also supplemented with a call for a "National Convention . . . for the elevation of the standards of medical education in the United States."

That convention met in May 1846, but because some participants felt that the attendance was not representative of the national profession, it adjourned after resolving to meet the following year with a plan for a permanent National Medical Association and with draft proposals for improvement of premedical and medical education and a code of medical ethics. That resolution was offered by Dr. Isaac Hayes of Philadelphia, who in the intervening year arranged a more representative meeting and ghosted the code that a committee of seven presented to the Second National Medical Convention, held in Philadelphia on May 5–7, 1847. *Ghosted* is the apt word because, in a prefatory note, Hayes (a modest man despite great attainments) stated that the code was framed largely in the words of Percival, with "a few sections in the words of the late Dr. Rush." Dr. Hayes was most probably the principal redactor of the document. His deep familiarity with the literature of medicine and medical ethics, and the marks of his own sympathies in wording and content, make the attribution reasonable.

Hayes erased from Percival's text the strong language of class distinctions more suited to the British setting and transformed Percival's "tacit compact" between the profession and society into a social contract with a set of mutual rights and duties among the profession, patients, and society as a whole. Dr. Rush's "few words" accomplished this transformation. Lifted from his lecture "On the Duties of Patients to their Physicians," they constitute the entire article II of the first chapter and bring something entirely new to Percival's conception of medical ethics. The list of duties is not unreasonable, yet the idea that physicians have "a right to expect and require that their patients should entertain a just sense of the duties which they owe to their medical attendants" puts medical ethics into a thoroughly American context.[17]

Dr. John Bell, chairman of the drafting committee, contributed an eloquent preface. Bell's words make this American philosophy explicit. After noting that "medical ethics, as a branch of general ethics, must rest on the basis of religion and morality. They comprise not only the duties, but, also, the rights of a physician," Bell continues in a philosophical vein, "every duty or obligation implies, both in equity and for its successful discharge, a corresponding right." Physicians have a duty to advise and a reciprocal right to be "attentively and respectfully listened to"; physicians have a duty to endanger their lives and health for the community's benefit and a reciprocal right to be protected from "the unnecessary exhaustion of their benevolent sympathies." All the physician's skills and talents are held "in trust for the public good." Bell firmly announces, "Medical ethics cannot be so divided as that one part shall obtain the full and proper force of moral obligations on physicians universally, and, at the same time, the other be construed in such a way as to free society from all restrictions in its conduct to them." He particularly repudiates the "caprice of the hour"—presumably the current Jacksonian egalitarianism—"to determine whether the truly learned shall be overlooked in favor of ignorant pretenders."[18] Here, then, medical ethics becomes in substance that very American political fiction, a contract with mutual rights and duties among the contracting parties: doctors, patients, and society. An intriguing idea but, in this context, an odd one: it is only the physicians who have written the contract.

Bell and his fellow drafters revised Percival's *Medical Ethics* to suit this new conception, radically modifying Percival's division of chapters to reflect their own philosophy of "tacit contract" and "reciprocal rights and duties." Percival's division into four chapters on duties of physicians in hospitals, duties in private practice, duties toward apothecaries, and duties relative to the law is reshaped into three quite different chapters. Chapter I is devoted to the duties of physicians to their patients and the obligations of patients to their physicians (here Rush is welded to Percival). Chapter II contains the duties of physicians to each other and to the profession. Chapter III covers the duties of the profession to the public and the obligations of the public to the profession. The Code of Ethics of the American Medical Association (as the new organization named itself) was, thanks to Bell and Hayes, a thorough translation of Percival's British into the American idiom.[19]

The first chapter of the Code of Ethics begins with a strong affirmation, "A physician should . . . be ever ready to obey the calls of the sick," and imposes obligations of "faithful attendance, confidentiality and consultation in difficult cases," followed by a list of the duties of patients. This chapter, despite its innovative format, contains little that cannot be found in the decorums and deontologies of the medical ethics tradition (even the duties of patients, which were delineated in the confessional books of the Middle Ages). However, Chapter II, "The Duties of Physicians to Each Other, and to the Profession at Large," was strikingly innovative in content. After some familiar words from the tradition urging respect for the profession and the attainment of "purity of character and high moral standards," physicians are issued instructions prohibiting advertising, patents on surgical instruments and medicine, secret nostrums, and urging free service to colleagues.

Article IV, "Of the Duties of Physicians in Regard to Consultations," lays down rules about the conduct of consultations and their etiquette, but one passage anchors the section:

> [A]s in consultations the good of the patient is the sole object in view, and this is often dependent on personal confidence, no intelligent regular practitioner, who has a license to practice from some medical board of known and acknowledged respectability, recognized by this association and who is in good moral and professional standing in the place in which he resides, should be fastidiously excluded from fellowship or his aid refused in consultation, when it is requested by the patient. But no one can be considered as a regular practitioner, or a fit associate in consultation, whose practice is based on an exclusive dogma, to the rejection of the accumulated experience of the profession, and of the aids actually furnished by anatomy, physiology, pathology and organic chemistry.[20]

The intent is obvious. The new AMA will "recognize" medical boards "of known and acknowledged respectability." Obviously, no such board would license practitioners "whose practice is based on an exclusive dogma," namely, homeopathy or Thomsonianism and their like (although "exclusive dogma" remains vague enough to include many an unacceptable doctrine). Such boards will, of course, license those who have studied and employ the medical sciences in their practice. This broad framework of education, licensure, and "recognition" surrounds the consultation. "Fit associates in consultation"—that is, physicians who should be called in or to whom a patient should be referred—will henceforth be not only those "in good moral and professional standing," but those who, in addition, meet the educational and regulatory standards of the new association.

Chapter II of the Code of Ethics, says a historian, "became the heart of the code and the source of the profession's subsequent troubles during the 19th century."[21] It was hoped that by restricting ethical consultation to members of the same medical society, or to those practicing only "scientific" medicine, the Code would become a weapon to drive irregular practitioners out of business. Instead, the restriction became a focus of contention within the regular profession: the AMA expelled the New York State Medical Society in 1882 because it had promulgated its own code allowing cooperation with homeopaths. Similar skirmishes took place constantly. One medical leader, disgusted with the wrangling, proclaimed, "we want an association in which there will be no medical police and no medical ethics!"[22] Thus, the AMA Code, although it inherited the decorum and deontology of the tradition, loudly proclaimed a new politic ethics for the profession. The profession would find its place in American society by becoming an educated and ethical profession and by excluding—and convincing the public to exclude—"irregular" practitioners, defined broadly as anyone "whose practice is based on an exclusive dogma." The Code's politic ethics generated mighty political battles for the rest of the century.[23]

The Code was widely praised. It was often eulogized in medical school commencement addresses. Dr. George Wood, president of the AMA in 1853, advised every physician to keep a copy for handy reference since, "next to Holy Scripture and the grace of God, it would serve most effectually to guard him from evil."[24] Prominent physicians such as Austin Flint and Nathan Smith Davis wrote extensive commentaries on its precepts.[25] Davis predicted that the prescriptions of the Code "will probably continue to be the guide of medical men through the centuries to come."[26] The Code also had its critics. Some found it banal and insulting, suited, as one said, for "Mother Goose Tales."[27] Other critics were even more cynical, noting that it failed to recognize that the relationship between doctor and patient was essentially a business in which the doctor was only half of a mercantile transaction governed by the laws of supply and demand: "This may be a humiliating view of our practical status in the community but it is undoubtedly the true one."[28]

Two years after the Code appeared, Dr. Worthington Hooker, a graduate of Harvard Medical School and Professor of Theory and Practice of Medicine at Yale, published *Physician and Patient or a Practical View of the Mutual Duties, Relations and Interests of the Medical Profession and the Community*.[29] Hooker's volume, perhaps more than any other American work of the nineteenth century, was a compendium of medical ethics as it was understood in that era. Lucidly written chapters are devoted to the appropriate relationships between physicians, to the physician's crucial role as a "cordial of hope" in serious illness, to truthfulness, and to the moral influence of physicians on their patients. Hooker's chapter on truth in intercourse with the sick argues that physicians have a moral duty never to deceive the sick. Using the panoply of arguments about truth-telling that moral philosophy textbooks of the time often mustered—deception is often transparent, undermines trust, and has damaging effects on the deceiver, the deceived, and society in general—Hooker undertakes to refute Percival's latitudinarian view that some circumstances justify deception for the patient's own good. Hooker disdains the casuistry about truth-telling and permits only that on some occasions truth may be withheld; falsehood may never be perpetrated. His arguments on this topic anticipate those of Richard Cabot half a century later.

Dr. Hooker's book outlines a decorum of sympathy, dedication, probity, and courtesy. He imposes a deontology of truth and confidentiality. However, the dominant message of the book is the importance of being an educated and rationally critical physician, committed to the facts as science and experience reveal them. From the opening chapter on the "Uncertainty of Medicine," through a detailed criticism of quackery, Thomsonianism, and homeopathy, to chapters on the criteria whereby good practice could be distinguished from bad practice and on the appropriate roles of theory and observation, Hooker extols the scientifically educated physician. His view coincides exactly with that of the AMA's founders: medicine must be put on a scientific basis, and its practitioners must be educated in the appropriate application of that basis to their practice. Hooker hopes that "the great object for which the association was formed, 'the elevation and advancement of our common calling,' will be rigorously and steadily prosecuted." An appendix to this book contains the AMA Code, "in which the reader will find concisely stated the rules and principles which I have endeavored to illustrate in this . . . work."[30]

Several chapters of *Physician and Patient* explore the logical and psychological sources of medical error: some physicians are so entranced by a particular approach as to become "one idea men"; many others fall into the fallacy *post hoc, ergo propter hoc*, seeing "whatever follows a cause as being the result of that cause."[31] These observations on clinical decision making, together with Hooker's views of the ethics of anesthesia, which we shall discuss later, anticipate the shift in ethics from an emphasis on character and decorum to closer attention to the actual process of decision making in clinical care.

Dr. Austin Flint, one of the most distinguished physicians of the post–Civil War era, vigorously defended the National Code. He had been a founder of the AMA and for most of his career served as Professor of Principles and Practice of Medicine at Bellevue Hospital in New York City. In 1883 he published a commentary on the National Code of Ethics entitled *Medical Ethics and Etiquette*. His "Introductory Remarks" begin by demonstrating that "the principles of duty applied to medicine constitute a distinct branch of ethical science, just as do public ethics and social ethics." There are rules of conduct regarding relationships with patients, such as discretion, confidentiality, the duties of charity, and so on that have "moral weight." Medical etiquette consists of formalities to be observed in professional intercourse that are matters of convention, without the binding force of ethical rules. A Code that states both the ethics and etiquette expected from the profession contributes "to the purity and dignity of the medical profession . . . and are of far more importance to the public welfare than to physicians."[32] Flint's commentary follows the chapters of the National Code, dealing with duties to patients, to colleagues, and to the public. With regard to the much debated issue of consultation with irregular practitioners, he takes the position, in sympathy with his New York colleagues, that physicians should judge their own duty in this regard. Rather than forbidding consultation outright, which may on occasion harm patients who are being treated by irregulars, he allows for some exceptions. Consultations may be appropriate when the irregular practitioner does not take a position antagonistic to the regular profession, believing that he alone knows the truth and that the regular profession is wrong and dangerous. Flint's work, with its strong emphasis on professional unity and public welfare, contributed to the politic ethics of the profession.

During the final quarter of the nineteenth century, vigorous debates raged around most of the Code's provisions in Chapter II. Dissent arose over patents on surgical tools; over whether fees should be set based on the duration of medical attendance, the degree of skill required, and the nature of the disease; over whether fees should be adjusted to patients' means; and over advertising. During most of this period, the contention over consultation with irregular practitioners that had compelled the nascent AMA to formulate the Code continued. Medical societies and emerging specialty groups were deeply divided over the extent to which their members could collaborate with persons whose training and theories differed from their own.[33]

It was not only training and theories that divided physicians: race and gender did also. In 1870, several well-qualified African-American physicians were refused membership in the Medical Society of the District of Columbia. They and their white supporters then formed the National Medical Society of the District of Columbia and, in May 1870, applied to be seated as an official delegation to the AMA convention. The disputed claim to represent the District of Columbia was referred to the Ethics Committee; several resolutions from the floor urged abolition of any discrimination against qualified physicians. As the meeting ended, Dr. Nathan S. Davis, a stalwart founder of the AMA, reported that although race had not been a consideration, the Ethics Committee recognized the credentials of the segregated group. From that time until the 1960s, African-American physicians were admitted only if their local medical society would admit them and, for the most part, this was rare; the AMA refused to reprove medical societies that persisted in discrimination.[34] The National Medical Association was founded in 1895 as the organizational home for African-American physicians, dentists, and pharmacists.

Organized medicine treated women physicians with similar disdain. From the day in 1849 that Dr. Elizabeth Blackwell graduated from Geneva Medical College as America's first formally educated woman physician, women found themselves marginalized in medicine. Male physicians argued that women were not suited psychologically or physically for medicine; that medicine was contrary to the female virtues; and that it was incompatible with their vocation as wives and mothers. A number of women's medical schools were founded because almost all existing schools refused to admit women. The Johns Hopkins Medical School opened its first class to women in 1893 only because a group of wealthy women conditioned their donations on admission of women. For those women who attained a medical education, hospital privileges were difficult to obtain, membership in medical societies was reluctantly granted, and women were formally admitted to the AMA only in 1915. Against all this opposition, a small number of women achieved notable success. Still, as Regina Morantz-Sanchez, historian of women in American medicine, writes, "No matter how successful individual and exceptional women physicians would be in integrating themselves into the male professional world . . . as a group women physicians remained poised around the edges of that world, making contributions that were socially useful but otherwise devoid of the flashy eclat which measured success by male professional standards."[35]

Toward the end of the nineteenth century, a bitter dispute arose over payment for referral of patients between physicians. As medicine had become more specialized, specialists who depended on general practitioners for referral of patients began to offer fees to those practitioners who sent them patients. Quickly recognized as potentially detrimental to patients, who might be referred to a specialist even if they had no medical need, the practice was branded by many as unethical. The American College of Surgeons, after long internal strife, endorsed this position in 1912.[36]

An equally contentious argument raged over *contract practice*, in which physicians contracted with businesses and fraternal organizations to provide medical service to employees or members for a per capita fee. Opponents of this practice claimed that it created a conflict of interest for the contracted physicians and put patients in danger of being underserved. Contract practice, of course, drew patients away from private physicians. Many medical societies expelled physicians who participated in contract practice, branding them as unethical. From the noble days of the promulgation of the Code down to the opening of the twentieth century, politic ethics dominated American medical life. The attempts to formulate guidelines, not so much about personal behavior but rather about medical policy preoccupied the ethical debates. What Thomas Percival had begun in Manchester, with his attempt to regulate the association of surgeons and physicians, became in America the primary focus of professional ethics.[37]

The growth of politic ethics that accompanied the struggle of regular medicine to establish itself as a profession did not dampen the deeper moral commitments of many American physicians. The preaching of moral rectitude was common in a nation where religion was taken very seriously. As doctors moved into positions of greater social respectability, they began to take responsibility for educating and enforcing the moral rectitude proper to the Christian person and to the Christian nation that they, and almost everyone else, believed the United States to be. "In both their public and private lives," notes one historian, "nineteenth century doctors viewed themselves as physicians of both body and soul . . . it was precisely this dual responsibility that demanded a Christian spirit in medicine. The healing art was to be administered with the idea of elevating every man to the final glory of the Redeemer's kingdom."[38]

This conjunction between medicine and religion was not, as we might think today, purely arbitrary. Much of the medical theory of the time linked health to moral rectitude. Dr. Rush had lectured on the "Influence of Physical Causes on the Moral Faculty," the capacity to distinguish between good and evil. He taught his students that poor diet, inadequate sleep, excessive drink, and uncleanliness could lead to "micronomia," a weakened moral faculty.[39] Dr. Bell's Introduction to the AMA Code had noted that "physicians are enabled to exhibit the close connection between hygiene and morals, since all the causes contributing to the former are nearly equally auxiliary to the latter."[40] Dr. Hooker had devoted a chapter in *Physician and Patient* to the "Moral Influence of Physicians." Reflecting on the intimate association between physicians and their patients, the esteem in which patients hold their doctors, and the frequency with which they seek their advice, Dr. Hooker exclaimed, "what responsibility then rests upon the physician! How careful should he be in the expression of his opinions! At what high ends should he aim in his daily example! How important that he should be right upon the great moral questions which agitate the community, and that his morality should be strictly that of the Bible!"[41]

Medical theory taught that basic physiology consisted in the conservation and proper distribution of vital forces or nervous energy; it was logical to believe that the behaviors usually stigmatized as immoral, such as drunkenness and sexual excess, dissipated those energies and caused illness. *Neurasthenia* was the popular disease of post–Civil War America: this dissipation of nervous powers was manifested in almost every symptom, from exhaustion and flushing to dyspepsia, headaches, and chills. Its treatment ranged from application of electricity to sexual continence, but almost every treatment and prescription involved a strong dose of morality, often focused on sexual mores. Depletion of sperm by masturbation or nocturnal emission was a primary cause of male neurasthenia; female neurasthenia was traced to sexual excitation, to social excitation evinced by wandering too far from the female role of mother and wife, and to physical constriction from corseting. The moral remedies prescribed sexual restraint and adherence to one's natural role in life. Even the medical advice against corseting took on a strongly moral tone, mixing medical views on the pathological effect of tight lacing on internal organs with warnings on the impropriety of false sexual attractiveness.[42]

Neurasthenia is, of course, only one example of the mixing of morals and medicine. Other comprehensive diagnostic categories, such as *intestinal toxicity*, linked pathophysiology to behavior that contravened nature's law, which was equally God's law. A reformed life of temperance in every respect was the best cure. The enormously popular "crusaders for fitness," William P. Alcott, Sylvester Graham (of Graham Crackers), and John Harvey Kellogg (of Corn Flakes), preached highly moralistic health messages. Alcott constantly reminded physicians that they must "impress upon the public the realization that illness is sin; it comes only from transgression of divine laws."[43] The medical world was strongly against contraception, believing that almost all contraceptive practices except continence were physically and psychologically damaging and, of course, made marriage, ordained by God for procreation, into a licensed opportunity for sexual pleasure. Throughout the second half of the nineteenth century, the leading medical journals announced scientific theses that were analogous to the moral imprecations declaimed from the pulpits of American churches. Medicine proved the value of morality; morality enhanced the prestige of medical advice. The historian of medicine Charles Rosenberg succinctly states the prevailing view of the nineteenth century:

> [M]ost nineteenth century physicians assumed that there could be no conflict between their findings and the truths of morality. The human organism was a thing both material and divine and offenses both physical and moral were punished by disease. Drinking, overeating, sexual excess, all carried with them inevitable retribution, not because the Lord deigned to intercede directly in human affairs but because He had created man's body so that infringing on God's moral law meant disobeying the laws of physiology. Moralism thus drew upon the prestige of science, while medicine was pleased that its findings supported the dictates of morality.[44]

Certainly not all medical men were committed believers. Indeed, it was not uncommon for the local doctor to also be the local freethinker. Dedicated to the physical, physicians lost a sense of the spiritual. Some, such as Dr. Woods Hutchinson, were outspoken critics of religion and advocates of a naturalistic, evolutionary ethic.[45] Yet, in a country where religion was highly esteemed, even skeptical practitioners might not want to advertise their skepticism. American physicians in the nineteenth century were satisfied with the conjunction of science and morals that modern medicine had become. They were pleased to assume the roles of moral arbiter and counselor. The AMA Code urged, "The opportunity which a physician not infrequently enjoys of promoting and strengthening the good resolutions of his patients, suffering under the consequences of vicious conduct, ought never to be neglected."[46]

Sexual immorality was often the "vicious conduct" that needed correction by good medical advice. Sexual morality was at the heart of another major moral question posed to American medicine and its public: should male physicians care for women in pregnancy and parturition? Male midwives had appeared in Europe and England in the seventeenth century; the medical specialty of obstetrics developed during the eighteenth century. Yet, female midwives continued to attend, as they had for centuries, at most births. Obstetricians were few, and most of them were professors. Physicians were summoned, when available, only in the direst emergencies. However, obstetricians and general practitioners gradually became the common attendants, in part because a powerful movement, fostered by organized medicine at the end of the nineteenth century, regulated midwives almost out of existence. However, the ascendancy of male obstetricians was not without moral controversy. As late as 1857, one writer could say, "the practice of man-midwifery is among the noxious weeds which the rank luxuriance of civilization has produced."[47] Physical examination of women by male physicians was considered offensive to female modesty and surrounded by stringent limitations. Textbooks on obstetrics advised that a "touching examination" be attended by a female friend of the patient, carried out in a darkened room with the patient clothed, and performed tactually rather than visually.[48]

In abortion, American physicians found a cause that enhanced both their reputation for moral responsibility and their professional standing. The English common law view that abortion should be considered criminal only after quickening prevailed in the United States. In 1821, Connecticut passed the first statute prescribing life imprisonment for anyone "who shall willfully and maliciously administer . . . any deadly poison . . . with an intention to cause or procure the miscarriage of any women then being quick with child."[49] Within the next 20 years, 14 other states passed similar statutes; several states, such as New York, added the phrase "unless the same shall have been necessary to preserve the life of such woman, or shall have been advised by two physicians to be necessary for that purpose."[50] These statutes were part of a general move to revise American civil and criminal law; they did not arise from any broad public concern about abortion and essentially made little difference in the legal view that had prevailed in Anglo-American jurisdictions for centuries.

During the 1840s, abortion came into view as a social problem. It appears that the incidence of abortion had risen dramatically. This procedure was sought largely by upper-class white Protestant women who desired to limit their childbearing. Abortions were frequently performed by abortionists, called *wise women* or *lady doctresses*, and by other irregular practitioners. Newspapers carried advertisements for abortifacients or consultation for "private female diseases." Sensational cases, such as that of the abortionist Madame Restell, who ran a large commercial abortion enterprise in New York, made the papers. In 1857, Dr. Horatio R. Storer, a Boston obstetrician and Harvard Professor of Obstetrics initiated a campaign to organize regular physicians against abortion and in favor of stricter law. Within two years he had generated enough support that the AMA, meeting in Louisville, Kentucky, resolved "publicly to enter an earnest and solemn protest against the unwarranted destruction of human life" and, recognizing the traditional duties of "its grand and noble calling, to urge the several legislative assemblies of the Union to revise abortion laws."[51] The revision most desired was the extension of criminality to the destruction of fetal life from conception, not just from the time of quickening (medical opinion considered quickening irrelevant), and the clear indictment of any procurer of abortion who acted without sound medical judgment that the abortion was necessary to save the mother's life. James C. Mohr, a historian of these events, concludes, "the vigorous efforts of America's regular physicians would prove in the long run to be the single most important factor in altering the legal policies toward abortion in this country."[52]

The doctors were ahead of the clergy, who only slowly and under the doctors' prodding took to the pulpit against abortion, often acknowledging the "medical profession's noble stand."[53] Three major denominations—the Congregationalists, the Presbyterians, and the Episcopalians—endorsed the medical campaign during the 1860s; American Roman Catholics reaffirmed their ancient opposition to abortion at the Tenth Council of Baltimore in 1869 (yet no Catholic newspaper noticed Pope Pius IX's condemnation in the same year!).[54] Most physicians, Catholic or Protestant, had a deep moral repugnance for abortion, and any woman seeking help was unlikely to get it from her doctor. However, American physicians clearly had self-interested motives in this movement. They were engaged in a serious attempt to drive irregulars out of practice and to achieve moral and legal standing in the land. Legal revision that recognized the importance of professional medical opinion powerfully advanced these motives.

In addition, the anti-abortion campaign arose from the genuine belief that abortion and the sexual license that it implied were moral evils that weakened the fabric of the nation's life. Mohr concludes, "The nation's regular doctors, probably more than any other identifiable group in American society during the nineteenth century, including the clergy, defended the value of human life per se as an absolute. . . . Lobbying [for abortion laws] became holy work for those physicians who believed that the United States was damning itself as a society by continuing to commit mortal sins on a massive scale without even realizing it. The theme of saving America from itself was a common leitmotif throughout the medical campaign against abortion after 1860."[55] The ancient Hippocratic injunction that "I will never give to a woman a pessary to cause abortion," taken for granted as a moral rule for many centuries, became a conspicuous part of American medical deontology. Indeed, it became part of the politic ethics of American medicine.

7

American Medicine
Science, Competence, and Ethics

The founders of the AMA hoped to encourage the education of physicians "in anatomy, physiology, pathology and organic chemistry."[1] In 1847 these medical sciences were, as one medical historian says, in "transition to a physiological synthesis."[2] That physiological synthesis was the convergence of descriptive anatomy with chemistry and physiology. Exciting work was being done in Europe. In Germany, Justus von Liebig was inventing organic chemistry, Johannes Müller was creating neurophysiology, and his student Theodor Schwann was formulating the cell theory. In that same year, Rudolf Virchow published the first issue of his *Archiv* which would record the evolution of the science of cellular pathology. In Paris, Claude Bernard was developing the field of experimental medicine. American physicians learned of the exciting work being done abroad and sometimes participated as students or colleagues in European laboratories, but little scientific work was being done at home.

In the year before the AMA Code was promulgated, a clinical innovation opened a promising field of medical science. It also opened an ethical debate that, perhaps more than any other ethical discussion of the nineteenth century, previewed the debates that transformed medical ethics in the mid-twentieth century. That innovation was surgical anesthesia, and the ethical debate was over its moral acceptability.[3] On October 16, 1846, Dr. John Collins Warren, America's preeminent surgeon, removed a tumor from the face of a patient whom Dr. William T. G. Morton, a dentist, had rendered unconscious by administering vapor of diethyl ether, which he called Letheon. Within months, surgeons throughout the world were experimenting with the innovation; within a year, nitrous oxide and chloroform had been added to the anesthetic armamentarium. But, as one practitioner noted five years later, "the blessing [of anesthesia] is not unalloyed."[4] Over the next decade, the problems of this mixed blessing were aired in the medical and public press. These problems ranged from the physical dangers accompanying administration of these substances to broader matters of medical theory, such as

81

the healing power of pain, and to deeper matters of theology, such as the role of pain in divine providence.

The physical dangers became quickly apparent. An 1848 AMA report noted that the high doses of anesthetic required for surgery induced "convulsions, prolonged stupor, high cerebral excitement . . . asphyxia . . . bronchitis, pneumonia, [and] inflammation of the brain," and death was not unknown.[5] It was clearly necessary to use these substances with great care, and meticulous attention to the selection of appropriate patients was advised. The broader matters of medical theory included ancient and modern views on the place of pain in the processes of disease and healing. It was widely held that pain was a stimulus that promoted wound healing and cure. Elimination of pain would, in the opinion of many competent physicians, retard and even prevent healing. Also, a major segment of the profession had become convinced that the heroic therapies of the past, massive bleeding and violent purging, should yield to the gentler *vis mediatrix naturae*, the healing power of nature, and they feared that painless surgery would perpetuate aggressive surgical practices.

In an America saturated with religious belief, theological themes could not be erased from the debate. Suffering was, in Christian belief, a punishment for sin and a stimulus for repentance. The text of Genesis (3.16) where God curses Eve, mother of all humankind, saying, "in sorrow thou shalt bring forth children," needed an exegesis that could render painless childbirth compatible with faith. Other issues crowded into the debate: ether had a reputation as an intoxicating drug at the time when the temperance movement, with strong medical support, was fighting intoxication. Anesthesia eliminated the patient's control over his or her operation; anesthesia gave the surgeon power over his patient. Anesthesia could provide an opportunity for medical immorality: within a year of the dramatic experiment in Boston, one medical paper announced an "alleged rape perpetrated on a female under the influence of ether."[6]

A variety of moral questions, then, attended this innovative technology. Over the next decade, however, the attraction of painless surgery to patients and physicians alike pressed the debate toward its acceptance, and its wide use during the Civil War rendered anesthesia more familiar. A powerful moral argument also helped carry the day: the values of humanitarianism that had gradually permeated American society. The abolition of torture and of slavery, concern for the welfare of animals, and alleviation of the suffering of the poor demonstrated that Enlightenment virtue had seeped into the once stern Calvinism of American culture. A God of mercy and love was being preached even from Calvinist pulpits. "Our every idea of a God of love and mercy constrains us to believe that He does not delight in the sufferings of his creatures," a physician could write in 1871.[7] Anesthesia emerged from the moral debate as a winner.

The medical historian Martin S. Pernick sees that debate as a profound revolution in medical morality. In the first half of the nineteenth century, many physicians adhered to the moral imperative that life should be saved at all costs, even by heroic and very painful means. Other physicians took a more gentle view of their art, believing that harm should be avoided even at the risk of failure to save life. "Heroic practitioners," Pernick writes, "regarded active intervention as the physician's primary ethical obligation; natural healers preferred to passively do no harm rather than risk causing harm directly. The heroic professional tradition encouraged risk-taking whenever a life might be saved; the ethics of natural healing sanctioned only safe and supportive therapies."[8] Pernick believes that the anesthesia debate fostered an intermediate position that he calls *conservative professionalism*. Leaders of the profession, such as Austin Flint, Worthington Hooker, and Valentine Mott, sought a mediating moral stance. It consisted of a utilitarian calculus that sought to balance the risks to be taken against the possible good to be achieved with any therapy.

An AMA committee report stated the position: "the great question, which still divides medical opinion, is: do the risks and evils attendant upon the use of these agents in surgery, counterbalance the advantages afforded by exemption from pain, and to what extent and under what circumstances is it proper to use them?"[9] This question seems very familiar to modern physicians and ethicists, yet at that time it was, according to Pernick, rather novel. The question had rarely been asked because the means of answering it were not available. Now the *numerical method* of statistics had entered medicine, providing a means of calculating the comparative results of treatment and nontreatment. "The prudent and judicious physician . . . calculates probabilities as accurately as he can at every step, and endeavors to make every measure tell upon the great result, avoiding, as far as possible, those which will not, and especially those which will hinder or defeat it," advised Dr. Worthington Hooker.[10] In the years following the introduction of anesthesia, many studies attempted the quantification of results that would allow physicians to do just that. And beyond that calculation was a new view of professional responsibility. The responsible physician was committed to making the right choice among many probabilities. It was possible to "synthesize the scientific and ethical conflicts racking the profession . . . to reduce morality to mathematics, to measure objectively whether the 'cure' or the 'disease' constituted the 'lesser evil'."[11]

If Pernick is correct, the anesthesia debate was the occasion for a revolution in medical morality that has persisted to our own time. It drew physicians away from broad metaphysical, theological considerations and from absolute moral commitments, and directed their attention toward a rational calculation of risks and benefits. Where that calculation led, the physician's therapeutic duty lay. At the same time, the anesthesia debate anticipated contemporary bioethics because it raised the broader metaphysical, theological, and theoretical questions about a new medical technology. But because the debate and its resolution were in the hands of the profession rather than in the domain of philosophers, theologians, and the public, it was resolved by a professional standard, albeit a novel one.

American medicine, therefore, was not unfamiliar with moral problems. Physicians, as well as the public, commonly acknowledged them. Yet, as medical historian Daniel Fox has said, there was an almost total "segregation between moral philosophy and medicine."[12] Many physicians, certainly all who had attended college, had studied moral philosophy, which was a required course for all college seniors. Many moral philosophers were familiar with medical theory and science; the most famous moral philosopher of the first half of the nineteenth century, Mark Hopkins, and the most famous in the second half, William James, had both studied medicine. Yet they rarely alluded to its problems in their philosophical writings.[13] There are glimpses of the style of early-nineteenth-century moral philosophy here and there in medical writing, as in John Bell's eloquent introduction to the original AMA Code. His statement that "every duty or obligation implies . . . a corresponding right" remotely reflects the treatise on "reciprocity" in Francis Wayland's popular text *Elements of Moral Science.*[14] Faint reminiscences of the Lockean social contract may tint the American revision of Percival.[15] Still, it seems correct to affirm that the influence of Percival on the medical profession narrowed the understanding of medical ethics to "questions about who shall practice medicine, in what relationship with other practitioners, and with what obligations to patients, institutions and public authority."[16] The more transcendent "elements" of moral philosophy and religion, on which Bell asserted that "medical ethics, as a branch of general ethics, must rest," faded far into the background.[17]

The etiquette in the relationship between physicians and their patients, and the relation of these parties to civil society that had dominated the medical ethics of the nineteenth century, began to shift as science gained authority in medical theory and practice. A pivotal moment came when Johns Hopkins University opened on September 12, 1876. One of the most popular moral philosophers of the English-speaking world, Thomas Henry Huxley, gave the principal address. Although that university's medical school was still almost two decades in the future, Huxley chose to speak of medical education. He celebrated the recent re-creation of medicine as a "branch of experimental physiology" and asserted that the aim of medical education was to inculcate sufficient science to be effective in diagnosis, therapy, and prevention. Effectiveness was the principal criterion of right medical conduct, a concept already adumbrated in Hooker's thought.[18] So it was that as one Englishman, Thomas Percival, stamped American medical ethics with his conception of a professional and gentlemanly code, another Englishman, Thomas Huxley, endorsed a new conception of professional competence.

This conception of professional competence provides the foundation for a view of medical ethics formulated by Dr. Richard C. Cabot (1868–1939). Cabot graduated from Harvard College, earned his medical degree at the Harvard Medical School, and then passed his entire career as a member of the Harvard faculty. In 1919 he was appointed Professor of Clinical Medicine in the Medical School and

Professor of Social Ethics at Harvard College. He was a highly respected clinician, and his books *Physical Diagnosis* and *Differential Diagnosis* went through many editions. He brought to perfection the case method in teaching medical students,[19] and he inaugurated the Clinical Pathological Conference at Massachusetts General Hospital in 1909. Acutely sensitive to the changes that American medicine was undergoing at the turn of the century, Cabot thought deeply about them: the shift of care to the hospital, the use of ancillary professions such as social work in caring for the patient, and the increasing appreciation of science in understanding disease.[20]

Dr. Cabot transformed himself into a respectable moral philosopher. A friend of such renowned philosophers as Josiah Royce, Ernest Hocking, and Ralph Barton Perry, he read widely and formulated his reflections into a systematic ethics. In his principal philosophical book, *The Meaning of Right and Wrong*, he analyzes "agreements, desires and needs" as the "stuff of ethics," proposing that "our all inclusive need is growth and I think we may make it fulfill the specifications of an authoritative aim in life." He argues that "right desires, agreements and plans are those that are governed by reality as it shows itself in our needs. Wrong desires, agreements and acts are those that diverge from reality and our needs through self-deceit."[21] In addition to being a competent amateur philosopher, Dr. Cabot was a devout Christian who wrote about the Christian life in general as "consecrating the affections" and about the duties of pastors in ministering to the sick.[22] Still, even as a philosopher and Christian, he formed a particularly modern view of medical ethics in the evolving world of medicine. Medical historian Chester Burns describes Cabot's place in that world:

> The all-purpose general practitioner of the nineteenth century—a Christian gentleman of intrinsic goodness, law abiding and loyal to the codified rules of one professional society—had been replaced by a new group of specialist practitioners . . . rooted in experimental science and elaborate methods of clinical evaluation and patterns of clinical care. . . . As much as any other physician of his day Richard Cabot demonstrated the validity of the new bases for professional goodness. . . . Whether or not the practitioner went to church on Sunday, knew the "Star Spangled Banner," swore the Hippocratic Oath, or adhered to precepts about consultation in the AMA Code of Ethics were not the important criteria for judging professional propriety. What counted [for Cabot] was whether a practitioner understood the specific diseases, their causes, signs, symptoms, courses, prognoses, treatments—and whether each practitioner applied this understanding in the assessment and management of each individual patient.[23]

In a short article titled "Medical Ethics in the Hospital," Cabot enumerated the duties of the modern physician working with others in the hospital setting.[24] Extensive cooperation between physicians and all other professionals involved in the care of patients was required. Accurate records of patient care must be kept and analyzed. The number of patients assigned to doctors must not be so great as to compromise attention to all patients. Patients should be informed of their diagnoses, and their treatments should be explained to them by their attending physicians. Patients should not be exploited for teaching purposes. Senior physicians should not exploit their junior colleagues, either by assigning them work they themselves should do or by taking credit for their scientific contributions. Disputes over appropriate care should be settled by committees. This list of ethical duties, remarkably different from the disquisition of Hooker, who himself had appreciated the scientific grounding for practice but whose mind remained largely in the mold of Hippocratic decorum, initiates what might be called "an ethic of competence."[25]

Since ancient times, physicians had been told that attaining knowledge and skill was a primary obligation, but throughout most of medical history, few methods for measuring knowledge and skill had been available. A memorized mastery of Galen's treatises had to suffice. As the medicine of the nineteenth century absorbed the advances in physiology, pathology, and bacteriology and learned to use the numerical method to evaluate the results of treatment, knowledge and skill became more measurable. Hooker's advice about balancing probabilities was, by Cabot's time, even more realizable. Cabot himself had analyzed 1000 consecutive autopsies at the Massachusetts General Hospital and had demonstrated a high rate of error in diagnosis. His publication of this analysis and a later similar study dismayed and angered many of his colleagues, who accused him of the ethical breach of "publicly advertising the faults of the general practitioner."[26] But for Cabot, this *was* ethics: moral practice was competent; incompetent practice was unethical. Clinical competence had moved to the center of medical ethics.

Clinical competence, in Dr. Cabot's view, was not a cold, calculating skill. It had to include not only mastery of science but also appreciation of the personal and social needs of the patient. Like his younger Harvard colleague Dr. Francis W. Peabody, Dr. Cabot understood and taught that "One of the essential qualities of the clinician is interest in humanity, for the secret of the care of the patient is in caring for the patient."[27] He recognized what we now call the *humanistic* qualities of the physician, not as mere decorations on clinical competence but as intrinsic to it. In his earliest venture into philosophy, *What Men Live By*, Cabot was prompted to reflect on the basic values, which he described as Work, Play, Love and Worship, by recalling "tough and ancient problems which came to me through the Social Service Department of Massachusetts General Hospital." In dealing with the distressed and the sick, "Someone must win the affection of each sufferer, penetrate the past and guide the future better."[28]

In *Training and Rewards of the Physician*,[29] Dr. Cabot complained that "the human side of medical practice" was ordinarily left out of medical education: "the preparedness for treating a human being as if he possessed a mind, affections, talents, vices and habits good and bad, as well as more or less diseased organs."[30] He urged medical students to develop this "psychical preparedness" by astute observation of experienced practitioners and by reading the great literature that describes *la comédie humaine*. Insight into the human condition aids immeasurably in diagnosis and care of the patient. In addition, patients thrust upon their doctor the "great life problems, urgent as a bleeding wound . . . not a week passes in the practice of the ordinary physician but he is consulted about one or more of the deepest problems in metaphysics and religion—not as a speculative enigma, but as part of human agony. It is one of the great rewards of medicine to be given the opportunity to help patients in this way."[31]

Dr. Cabot took a forthright stand in the long debate over medical truth-telling. Early in his medical career he wrote an article on the topic, and at the end of his career as an ethics professor, he wrote an entire book on honesty. He opened *Honesty* with the words "For at least half a century, I have found honesty a most interesting subject. Next to food and shelter it seems to be one of our greatest needs. . . . Yet we do not behave as if between men we valued honesty supremely. In medicine and in social work I have been amazed at the degree of acquiescence in dishonesty."[32] In his 1903 article "Truth and Falsity in Medicine," he had argued that, contrary to the prevailing ethic, patients should be told the truth about their diagnosis, prognosis, and treatment. He begins the article, as one would expect from a man impressed by the scientific method, by stating that he will argue for that thesis not by "metaphysical analysis" but by an experimental method, comparing as rigorously as possible the results of honest disclosure with those of dissembling. He calls on his own experience as a clinician and on that of other clinicians to demonstrate that "I have not yet found any case in which a lie does not do more harm than good."[33] Truth-telling enhances confidence and understanding between the physician and the patient. Truth-telling, said Richard Cabot, is a matter of "professional ethics" and, as such, is intrinsic to clinical competence.[34]

The truth-telling debate continued throughout the first several decades of the twentieth century. In 1927 a frequent writer on medical ethics, Dr. Joseph Collins, published the article "Should Doctors Tell the Truth?" in *Harpers*. He wrote, "the longer I practice medicine the more I am convinced that every physician should cultivate lying as a fine art. But there are many varieties of lying."[35] In contrast to Richard Cabot, he argued that the truth often caused harm. He offered as proof personal examples that contradicted the examples Cabot had provided. Physicians, said Dr. Collins, must make a utilitarian calculus to determine, as honestly as they can, when deception contributes more to a patient's welfare than does the truth. Collins was arguing with Cabot just as Hooker had argued with Percival and Percival with Gisborne. For all these men, anecdotes were the test. Although Dr. Cabot had claimed that his position was based on scientific experiments, his research consisted of well-organized anecdotes.[36]

Despite Richard Cabot's dedication to serious moral philosophy, he did little to draw philosophical ethics and medical practice together. He never wrote a systematic study of medical ethics. Beyond his insistence on competence as a moral imperative and his rather novel approach to truth-telling, his treatment of various ethical issues is rather casual. He touches on topics such as abortion, contraception, and euthanasia but does not take them much further than the conventional views. He stresses the traditional qualities of medical decorum, such as courtesy, fidelity, and patience, and believes that these qualities are best learned by osmosis from medical chiefs who are moral men. He says almost nothing that would contradict the standard paternalistic ethic of the time.[37] Still, Cabot stands at an important turning point in American medicine when scientific medicine had taken firm hold and when it was reasonable to insist that the practitioner's highest moral duty was to master that scientific medicine for the benefit of the patient.[38]

The most admired physician in American and English medicine, William Osler (1849–1919), said little about the ethics of medicine. He was, of course, the constant proponent of medical competence and, in his prolific writings, gave sage advice about how physicians should live, study, and deal with their patients. However, he rarely rose to the level of high principle, being satisfied with simple rules. He stated:

> I have three personal ideals. One, to do the day's work well and not to bother about tomorrow. . . . The second ideal has been to act the Golden Rule, as far as in me lay, toward my professional brethren and toward the patients committed to my care. And the third has been to cultivate such a measure of equanimity as would enable me to bear success with humility, the affection of friends without pride and to be ready when the day of sorrow and grief came to meet it with the courage befitting a man.[39]

Although Osler's ethical teachings were *obiter dicta*, his personality and his reputation made him an ethical icon for generations. He prized above all the characteristic he called *equanimity*, "imperturbability . . . coolness and presence of mind under all circumstances, calmness amid storm, clearness of judgement in moments of grave peril, immobility, impassiveness or, to use an old and expressive word, phlegm. It is the quality that is most appreciated by the laity though often misunderstood by them."[40] Osler's address, delivered to the graduating class of the University of Pennsylvania School of Medicine in 1889, was bound into a small book, titled *Aequanimitas*, that became a favorite gift for graduating medical students for decades. It set a pattern for Anglo-American physicians of the early twentieth century: composed, even of temper, considerate, calm, and cautious. Thus, Osler's prestigious patronage gave maximum support to the Hippocratic advice that physicians perform their tasks "calmly and adroitly." This decorum, exemplified by "the most beloved physician of all time," was based on the simplest of deontologies, the Golden Rule and "the high moral ideals expressed in that most memorable of human documents, the Hippocratic oath."[41] Whether the veneration of Osler was justified or not, it left an almost indelible mark on medical ethics: ethics is what my best teacher does. This *role model* theory of ethics, impoverished as it is as an articulation of ethical responsibilities, particularly in difficult situations, acquired great popularity in the medical world. And as Dr. Osler's image faded, his place was taken by respected professors of medicine across the land.

In 1900, an event transformed the image of the physician from compassionate healer to hero. Drs. Walter Reed, James Carroll, Jesse Lazear, and Aristide Agramonte initiated a research program to determine the exact cause of Yellow fever, a disease that devastated the inhabitants of tropical countries. Under the sponsorship of the Surgeon General of the United States, the four physicians established a camp at Quemados, Cuba, where they exposed themselves (with the exception of Major Reed, who was away from the site) to the bites of one suspected agent, the mosquito. Dr. Lazear was infected and soon died. The experimenters then sought volunteers from among the American soldiers stationed there and local residents. Within several months conclusive proof was found that mosquito bites transferred the disease from person to person. Their discovery, which led to major public health initiatives in the affected localities, was widely hailed as both personal heroism and scientific achievement. The experimenter-physician took on heroic stature.

That celebrated event rose to the surface in a sea of ethical troubles: the scientific progress that medicine was enjoying was the result of a multitude of experiments with human subjects, most often patients and very often unknowing and unwilling objects of study. There was no clear direction in the long tradition. For centuries, the very word *experimentum* was the designation for any therapeutic attempt, and physicians commonly believed, in the words of Sir William Osler, that "every treatment is an experiment." At the dawn of the age of modern experimental medicine, one of its pioneers, Claude Bernard, wrote, "It is our duty and right to perform an experiment on man whenever it can save his life, cure him or gain him some personal benefit. The principle of medical and surgical morality, therefore, consists in never performing on man an experiment which might be harmful to him to any extent, even though the result might be highly advantageous to science, that is, to the health of others." This noble ethic did not inspire some medical scientists, who perpetrated outrageous experiments on patients who were often impoverished and ignorant. Even high-minded researchers found clinical material among the dying, whom, they judged, could not be harmed by their invasive studies. This poverty of ethical standards persisted until medical science worldwide was jolted into awareness by the Nazis' criminal adventures in medical research, which are related in a later chapter. American medical science was similarly jarred into serious reflection by the revelations that children, elderly patients, and poor African-Americans had been unconsenting subjects of harmful experiments. Not until the mid-1960s was the long tradition supplemented by an explicit ethic governing research with human subjects.[42]

Chauncey D. Leake has been called the "elder statesman of medical ethics."[43] Dr. Leake (1896–1978) may deserve the accolade, but he had nothing of the stuffy dignity of an elder statesman. He was not only a scientist but also a poet and a playwright, and he loved to argue about anything that fell within the ken of his capacious intellect. Trained as a pharmacologist, he and his team at the University of California Medical School during the 1930s produced significant research on anesthetic drugs, morphine antagonists, and amphetamines. He was a committed self-experimenter, always the first "human animal" on which new compounds were tried, sometimes with nearly fatal results.[44] This careful and creative scientist was also an ebullient humanist. He spoke several languages. He also published an edition of Egyptian medical papyri.[45] He read literature of extraordinary breadth. While serving as Chancellor of the Texas Medical Branch in Galveston, Dr. Leake printed a weekly broadsheet entitled "Calling to Your Attention," which contained brief reviews of 20 or 30 books or articles in science, medicine, history, philosophy, biography, and whatever else caught his attention. He was particularly interested in a problem that, in the 1930s, was frequently on the agenda of scientific convocations: the relation between science and other forms of knowledge.[46]

Chauncey Leake's interest in ethics was aroused early in his academic life. His Princeton mentor, the well-known moral philosopher Warner Fite, offered "delightfully informal preceptorials" that stimulated young Leake's eager mind.[47] As a graduate student in pharmacology at the University of Wisconsin, he did a research project on the Kappa Lambda Society of Aesculapius, the nineteenth-century secret medical society, sworn to uphold Percival's *Medical Ethics*. This led him to study Percival's own work. He wrote an article for the *Journal of the American Medical Association* on Percival's influence on medical ethics, and over the next few years he expanded that article into a new edition of the book that had had a pervasive effect on American medical ethics.[48]

Chauncey Leake was not a physician. He was a medical scientist who worked in constant collaboration with physicians and was a friendly critic of their ways. Strangely enough, Leake's interest in Percival was a negative one: while he admired much in the Manchester physician's writings, he judged that Percival had misconceived medical ethics from the beginning. He (unfairly, we now know) accused Percival of ignoring the philosophical literature on ethics and therefore of elaborating an "etiquette" rather than an "ethic," a sort of "Emily Post guide to proper professional conduct." Leake begins his prefatory essay to his edition of Percival with the remark, "The term 'medical ethics,' introduced by Percival is really a misnomer. Based on Greek traditions of good taste and on Percival's gentlemanliness, it refers chiefly to the rules of etiquette developed in the profession to regulate the professional contacts of its members with each other. . . ." Leake maintained that medical ethics must be more: it must be concerned with the ultimate consequences of the conduct of physicians toward their individual patients and toward society as a whole. The distinction between etiquette and ethics did not originate with Leake. He found it in W. H. S. Jones' 1924 monograph *The Doctor's Oath*.[49] Leake, however, thought of himself as the popularizer of the distinction. He remarked in the preface to the second edition, "Currently there seems to be clear recognition of the difference between medical etiquette and significant medical ethics. Yet fifty years ago I went a long way to emphasize the distinction."[50] In his view, this error had infected the American view of professional ethics.[51]

Dr. Leake insisted that professional ethics must be rebuilt on a foundation of moral philosophy. In an article that appeared the year after his volume on Percival, he sketched the ideal ethics course for medical students. The course should open with three lectures on the chief questions of moral philosophy, given by a member of the philosophy faculty, followed by a historical survey of ethics in medicine and then by an "informed discussion of actual case reports in medical ethics, referred to older, experienced, respected practitioners and debated actively with the students."[52]

Dr. Leake had a catholic view of moral philosophy: he always spoke of "the ethics" rather than "ethics" to make it clear that, in the course of human history, many different foundations for the moral life had been proposed. Over the years he built a long list of these ethics, which always began with "Pleasing the Big Boss" (an ethics of divine command, which he delighted to impugn as the source of patriarchy and misogyny). The long list was eventually refined to a short list of hedonism, social idealism, harmony, utilitarianism, pragmatism, and survival ethics.[53] Yet, behind these ethics, Leake glimpsed a more fundamental basis for the moral life. On July 3, 1939, he had a "Cartesian illumination" in the pleasant coolness of a redwood grove in the Santa Cruz Mountains. He had repaired there with his colleague from the University of California at San Francisco, Otto Guttentag (also a distinguished contributor to medical ethics), and several other scientists after a meeting of the American Association for the Advancement of Science. After Dr. Guttentag spoke on the influence of German and French philosophers on biological science, the group debated the popular question of a biological basis for ethics, a favorite topic of savants of the day. They concluded that "the probability of survival of a relationship between individuals or groups of individuals increases to the extent to which that relationship is mutually satisfying." This insight showed Leake the foundation for all of the ethics.[54]

Leake continued to write on the general topic of ethics in medicine and on specific issues in the field. He offered his views on human experimentation, organ transplantation, hemodialysis, and genetic control in his unique way, showing how one could adopt different positions on these topics, depending on which of the ethics one espoused. In his later years, he was an incessant and exuberant commentator on things medical and social. He vocally opposed the "hippyism" that flowed through his campus in the Haight-Ashbury district of San Francisco, which influenced, much to his dismay, the garb and lifestyles of the medical students. From 1974 until his sudden death in 1978, each Tuesday at noon, he lectured to a large audience of lunching students on "Practical Philosophy: the Ethics, the Logics, the Aesthetics." Those lectures were an entertaining trip through Dr. Leake's mind, as well as the world of science and medicine. Dr. Leake's last book, entitled *Practical Philosophy*, described "thirty well-formulated theories of ethics." He complained that "none of the professional philosophers who express concern about 'medical ethics' have paid any attention to it."[55]

Chauncey Leake was a somewhat idiosyncratic but prescient pioneer of modern medical ethics. In 1928 he wrote:

> Changing conditions in medical practice are making the matter [of teaching medical ethics] acute. It is becoming apparent that group practice, health insurance and periodic health examinations, as well as various aspects of public health measures, are profoundly altering the view of the physician. When it becomes financially more interesting for him to keep his patients well than to treat them when they are sick, the fundamental idealism of the medical profession will have a better chance to express itself, for the hedonistic consequences of the present financial system would not be so likely to follow.[56]

Those 70-year-old words preview current concerns about the ethical effects of managed care, anticipatory genetic diagnosis, and control of human immunodeficiency virus infection. These problems need more than etiquette for a solution. Which of the ethics can provide a solution remains a major question in the modern ethics of medicine that Dr. Leake envisioned.

Richard Cabot was a devout Christian; Chauncey Leake was a nonmilitant agnostic. Yet both men were intensely interested in ethics, and their ethical positions were not notably different. They stood in the American tradition of seeing growth as a fundamental good and, in Cabot's words, "an authoritative aim in life." Dr. Cabot did not bring to his views of medical morality any strong notes from his religious dedication, although he did collaborate with a minister, Rev. Russell Dicks, in writing *The Art of Ministering to the Sick* to educate pastors in caring for the sick.[57] Yet the link between religion and ethics continued to influence medical morality, although the religious and moral fervor of nineteenth-century American physicians had been submerged (but not drowned) in the tide of scientific professionalism and secularism that had swept over the United States in the 1920s and 1930s. By mid-century American medicine had become officially agnostic. The influence of theological ideas on medical theory had completely faded; overt religiosity had been banished from the doctor's consulting room. Physicians avoided inquiring into their patient's religious allegiance and feelings, and patients rarely knew their doctor's faith. Except for islands of denominational exclusiveness, such as Roman Catholicism and Orthodox Judaism, where doctrinal imperatives had to be honored even in medical care, the cathedrals of scientific medicine that were being erected in the nation's cities were empty of explicit signs of religious faith.

At the same time, the halls of those institutions were inhabited by many doctors and patients who went to church and thought religion a matter of importance in their lives. The concern about morality that religion has cherished can be translated into articulate expressions of ethical reasoning and analyses of moral problems. Roman Catholic theologians have had long experience with that sort of translation. In the United States, as a Catholic-sponsored health care system grew to significant proportions, theologians provided Catholic doctors, nurses, clerics, and patients with guides to doctrinally correct thinking about issues in medicine. One of the first of these, Father Charles Coppens' *Moral Principles and Medical Practice: The Basis of Medical Jurisprudence*, appeared in 1897. Coppens presented ethical arguments and church teaching on such issues as abortion, eugenics, euthanasia, and the therapeutic use of hypnosis. Other theologians authored similar works, culminating in the authoritative essays of Father Gerald Kelly during the 1950s, most of which were commentaries on the Ethical and Religious Directives adopted by the Catholic Hospital Association in 1948.[58] Even though these works reflected a particular doctrinal view, the ethical analyses were often expressed in rational terms that had broader appeal. As was noted in Chapter 4, distinctions with medieval roots, such as that between ordinary and extraordinary, continued to help physicians—Catholic, Protestant, and Jewish—understand complex moral questions.

Although outside Catholicism the analysis of medico-moral problems using the views and vocabulary of religious ethics was not widespread, interest was growing. In the same year that Cabot and Dicks published *The Art of Ministering to the Sick*, Dr. George Jacoby produced *Physician, Pastor and Patient. Problems in Pastoral Medicine.*[59] This non-denominational book discussed issues on which all pastors, physicians, and patients might seek enlightenment: abortion and contraception, suicide, divorce, sterilization, sex education, euthanasia, professional secrecy, and the treatment of "mental unfortunates." In each section, various arguments are exposed and a mediating conservative position is espoused.

The Dean of the Harvard School of Divinity, Willard Sperry, contributed to this growing literature. His book, *The Ethical Basis for Medical Practice*, resulted from an invitation from Dr. James Means, Chief of the Medical Service at Massachusetts General Hospital (MGH), who had asked Dean Sperry to give a talk to the medical staff.[60] Means explained that he, his faculty colleagues, and his house officers had been encountering problems that were in the realm of moral philosophy rather than medicine. Dr. Means sent Dean Sperry a typical case: a patient whose condition was hopeless suffered severe hemorrhaging that threatened to exhaust the MGH's supply of Rh negative blood. Sperry discusses the case in three chapters of his book and concludes that the patient's care should be predicated on the importance of the individual, as set down in the AMA Code. A physician must stay by the patient even though he knows he can do little or nothing for the patient. Sperry never addresses the problem of allocation of a scarce resource, nor does he ask about the patient's own preferences. He feels that the traditional values of the profession provide adequate guidance. Dr. Means, however, remarks in his preface that Dean Sperry may be too generous in his view of the profession. Medical historian Howard Vanderpool says of Sperry's pioneering contribution, "Sperry's book represents the values of many conscientious physicians in the late 1940s and 1950s because, like them, his view of medical morality was based on taking oaths and codes at face value. He believed that the medical profession practiced according to the highest professional standards which were rooted in the conscience, the sense of right and wrong in each individual."[61] Still, in a minor way, Dean Sperry was a pathbreaker in the literature of medical ethics: he was one of the first nonphysicians, and one of the first theologians, to contribute to a literature that had been the almost exclusive domain of physicians.

At almost the same time Sperry was lecturing to the medical staff at MGH, across the Charles River Joseph Fletcher was presenting the lectures that would become the first major contribution of a theologian to the new medical ethics that would be known as *bioethics*. Fletcher, a professor of moral theology at the Episcopal Theological School in Cambridge, had been invited to present the Lowell Lectures at Harvard University in 1949. Although he had not previously addressed moral issues in medicine (he had been deeply involved in social justice questions), he believed that medical ethics had been neglected by moralists and eagerly devoted his attention to problems of conscience in medical care. His lectures touched on the traditional topics of medical ethics: the right of patients to truth from their doctors, contraception, sterilization and euthanasia, and a relatively new problem, artificial insemination. Fletcher surveyed the traditional opinions about these problems, drawn from professional writings and from the one group of theologians who had addressed them, the Roman Catholics. Although the topics are relatively conventional, Fletcher gave them a turn that was revolutionary: he affirmed that in all these problems, it was the patient who had the right to decide what should be done. It was not the physicians or the church that held authority over the body and mind of the patient. He stated:

> [W]e shall attempt, as reasonably as may be, to plead the ethical case for our human rights (certain conditions being satisfied) to use contraceptives, to seek insemination anonymously from a donor, to be sterilized, and to receive a merciful death from a medically competent euthanasiast.[62]

This shift of authority from the duty of the doctor to the rights of the patient was a dramatic and crucial move toward a new medical ethics. The bioethics that would emerge some 20 years after the Lowell Lectures was built around the concept of the autonomy of the patient. Fletcher's contribution to the new medical ethics was seminal and for the next three decades he wrote vigorously about most of its topics. Fletcher, who transformed himself from theology professor to professor of medical ethics at the University of Virginia, was widely popular in medical circles.[63]

Physicians had assumed a professional persona that was shaped by an appreciation of scientifically dictated duties and that was noncensorious about their patients' moral or religious lives. The classic decorum described in the Hippocratic books, and repeated down the centuries, still suited the American doctor, with the addition of moral neutrality. The traditional admonitions about modest and neat dress were implemented by the adoption of the white coat that, says medical historian James C. Whorton, was borrowed from the laboratory to signify the clinician's dedication to science.[64] The deontology of the profession had been reduced to a concept of fiduciary responsibility, a concept shaped by the common law that required all professionals to serve their clients' interests rather than their own. The concept of fiduciary responsibility applied as much to lawyers, architects, and accountants as to physicians, but its superficial similarity to the Hippocratic injunction to help and not to harm allowed it to serve as the first principle of modern medical deontology. Almost the only other deontological principle was confidentiality, which, in the minds of many physicians, was an exceptionless rule.

Another rule of the old deontology lingered in ghostly form: the duty to provide free care for the sick poor. The long tradition, particularly in the Middle Ages, had insisted on this duty. The first and second editions of the AMA Code took it for granted, saying, "there is no profession, by the members of which eleemosynary services are more liberally dispensed than the medical. . . ."[65] The 1912 revision makes the duty explicit: "The poverty of a patient and the mutual professional obligation of physicians should command the gratuitous services of a physician."[66] The 1957 revision passes over this duty in silence. Many good doctors had incorporated that duty into their work. In its most prestigious form, the duty was fulfilled by a doctor guiding medical students during their clinical education without taking a fee. In a less prestigious way, doctors often dispensed with fees from those patients whom they knew to be hard pressed. Some physicians served without pay for one day each week in public hospitals. Little notice was given, however, to the multitudes of potential patients whose poverty prevented them from even approaching a physician. When health insurance became common after World War II, and when Medicaid and Medicare were initiated in the 1960s, charity medicine disappeared and the old deontology of gratuitous care for the poor faded from the physician's ethic.

A few other remnants of deontology could be found in the AMA Code, but they became fainter as the Code underwent successive revisions. The expansive Percivalian Code of 1847 had been revised in 1903 under the new name *Principles of Medical Ethics*. It was revised again in 1912, and with each revision it became briefer and less rhetorical. Dr. Rush's section on the duties of patients disappeared in 1903, together with the most restrictive language on consultation with irregulars. In 1957 a major revision cut the *Principles* down to ten terse statements reminiscent of the model of all deontological codes, the Mosaic Decalogue. The first statement of the shortened *Principles* is a somewhat rhetorical version of the doctrine of fiduciary responsibility: "Physicians must merit the confidence of those entrusted to their care, rendering to each a full measure of service and devotion."[67] Expressed in the most general terms, the *Principles* urge physicians to respect the rights of their patients, to keep up their skills, to accept the discipline of the profession, to consult when necessary, to keep confidences, and to be good citizens. They also forbid physicians to practice in circumstances where their independent medical judgment might be restricted or to obtain professional income other than remuneration for their services. The *Principles* are a relic of deontology: they are stated in a quasi-imperative, aphoristic form that directs physicians to act or avoid acting in certain ways. However, despite a prefatory reference to "the highest moral standards," it is clear that the *Principles* "are not laws [but] standards by which a physician may determine the propriety of his own conduct." This proviso takes the obligatory force out of any deontology, turning the Ten Commandments into the Ten Recommendations. In 1980 the *Principles* were revised again "to update the language, eliminate reference to gender and to seek a proper and reasonable balance between professional standards and contemporary legal standards."[68] That balance required the removal of the infamous "exclusive dogma" clause and one other principle that seemed to contradict federal laws against restraint of trade. The ten principles shrank to seven.

The tumultuous politic ethics of medicine had settled into tranquility. The wars of consultation and competition had been won. The medical marketplace was being allotted to the new specialties, state licensure laws were back in force and specialty certification was emerging, hospitals were largely under the control of their medical staffs, and contract and group practices were rare anomalies. Above all, twentieth-century physicians had attained the respectability and social authority that their nineteenth-century predecessors yearned for. Along with that respectability came enhanced income. By midcentury, the words Dr. Cabot had written in 1918 were no longer true: "Among the rewards which the doctor must not expect is wealth. . . . I have known few physicians fail to get a living in medicine, but the number who make comfortable incomes is equally few."[69] In just a few decades, American physicians had moved from being solid members of the middle class with moderate incomes to upper-class high earners. The aims of politic ethics—to organize medicine into a profession that merits public respect, commands authority in society, and guarantees a good living—seemed to have been achieved.[70]

Professional decorum, now surrounded with the aura of science, satisfied the public that doctors were decent, responsible, and competent. The deontology of fiduciary duty inspired trust. Popular literature in the United States had generally treated doctors more gently than had bitter European satires. American physicians were often portrayed as moral heroes. Sinclair Lewis' 1925 novel *Arrowsmith*, while critical of the profession's ignorance and venality, eulogized an idealistic young physician torn between a scientific career and the care of the poor. Two hit plays in the Broadway season of 1933–1934, *Men in White* and *Yellow Jack*, showed American doctors as "embodying the virtues of independence, integrity and dedication, even patriotism, in the service of the American public."[71] Dr. Kildare, appearing first in a 1936 short story, then in a popular film, and finally in a television series, was a competent and altruistic physician, beloved by millions of would-be patients, and the kindly Dr. Christian was family doctor to the nation.[72]

At midcentury, then, medical ethics as decorum, deontology, and politic ethics seemed settled. The principles and duties were known and acknowledged. The professional virtues were accepted and practiced, sometimes sincerely, sometimes pragmatically. Unquestionably, there were cheats, scoundrels, and fakes within the profession, and there were doctors whose ethics were the playacting of profiteers. But these could hide behind the stolid reputation of the majority of the profession. The place of medicine in society was firm. Medical ethics was communicated to young doctors by the example of their elders, rather than in lectures and courses. Few challenges to this settled state seemed apparent, and medical ethics became something of a backwater in the American medical world. Events, however, were to propel medical ethics to the center of attention.

8

A Chronicle of Ethical Events
1940s to 1980s

The sedate tradition of medical ethics was stirred into action in the decades after World War II. The biomedical sciences that had been making steady progress during the first half of the twentieth century rushed ahead during the war. The Committee on Medical Research (CMR), established by President Franklin D. Roosevelt in 1941, was charged with coordinating the work of medical scientists across the country with a view toward a more effective military medicine. The research sponsored by the CMR seized the advances of prior decades and rapidly directed them toward innovations in the prevention, diagnosis, and treatment of disease. The diseases that plague armies were the focus of attention: infection and battlefield wounds. This intense research spilled over into every realm of medicine. Between 1945 and 1965, antibiotic, antihypertensive, antipsychotic, and cancer drugs came into common medical use; surgery entered the heart and the brain; organ transplantation was initiated; and life-sustaining mechanical devices, the dialysis machine, the pacemaker, and the ventilator were invented. Into the hands of doctors came the most powerful weapons against disease and death that medicine had ever possessed. The weapons were not, however, unmixed blessings. Patients sometimes lingered in diminished condition. Deciding how to apply scarce technical resources, whether antibiotics or dialysis machines, proved agonizing. The scientific search for answers pressured researchers to turn patients into guinea pigs. The insights into the biology of reproduction and genetics that promised control over human procreation also raised fears of eugenics. The presence of machines by the bedside and the growing complexity of medical practice made the doctor's work more efficient but overshadowed the intimate and trusting association between doctor and patient.

The ambiguous nature of the medical miracles did not escape thoughtful scientists. During the 1950s, scientific and medical gatherings were occasionally devoted to examining this perplexing problem. One of those conferences began with the statement that "the world was unprepared socially, politically and ethically for the advent of nuclear power. Now biological research is in a ferment, creating and promising methods of interference with 'natural processes' which could destroy or could transform nearly every aspect of human life which we value. It is necessary for . . . every intelligent individual of our one world to consider the present and imminent possibilities."[1]

A series of events dramatized the scholars' questions and pushed the tradition of medical ethics to its limits. Some of these events are chronicled here, in the form of headlines with short news stories. Headlines are appropriate because all of these events made headlines when they occurred. However, the news stories expanded into a broad discourse of criticism, comment, and analysis. Some of this discourse was created by scientists and physicians, but much more was the work of philosophers, theologians, legal scholars, and social scientists. Some of this discourse was translated into health policy and health law, and often changed health care practices and institutions. The discourse led to a new medical ethics that came to be called *bioethics*.[2]

August 19, 1947: The Doctors' Trial at the Nuremberg Tribunal

In Nuremberg, Germany, on August 19, 1947, 20 Nazi physicians and three medical administrators, charged with "murders, tortures and other atrocities committed in the name of medical science," stood to hear the verdict delivered by the presiding judge of the War Tribunal convened by the victorious Allies to judge Nazi war criminals. These defendants had been charged with subjecting unwilling victims to medical procedures that were loosely called *scientific experiments*, thereby having caused their death, disfigurement, or disability. Nine of the defendants were sentenced to long prison terms, and seven were sentenced to death by hanging.

The Tribunal's verdict asserted that the evidence had shown that, "Beginning with the outbreak of World War II, criminal medical experiments on non-German nationals, both prisoners of war and civilians, including Jews and 'asocial' persons, were carried out on a large scale in Germany and the occupied countries." The Tribunal acknowledged that "certain types of medical experiments . . . conform to the ethics of the medical profession generally" and went on to delineate ten "basic principles that must be observed in order to satisfy moral, ethical and legal concepts." These ten points have become known as the Nuremberg Code.[3]

The first words of the Code state, "The voluntary consent of the human subject is absolutely essential. This means that the person involved . . . should be so situated as to be able to exercise free power of choice without the intervention of any element of force, fraud, deceit, duress, overreaching or any other ulterior form of constraint or coercion." The formal legal words veil the horror of the concentration camps in which these experimental subjects, totally stripped of their freedom and dignity, were mutilated and murdered under the guise of scientific research. The second norm, "the experiment should be such as to yield fruitful results for the good of society," directs the research to a human good rather than to the aims of an ideology. Subsequent principles require prior experiments with animals, the avoidance of unnecessary physical and mental suffering and injury, the assurance that no death or disabling injury will result, and scientifically qualified researchers. Researchers have the duty to terminate harmful experiments, and subjects have the right to withdraw from any experiment.

The "crimes committed in the guise of scientific research," as the prosecution's brief described the Nazi experiments, violated all of those principles. High-altitude research deprived victims of oxygen until they died. Persons were slowly frozen to death. More than 1000 persons were infected with malaria and treated with various experimental drugs: many died from the disease and many others from drug complications. Persons were infected with jaundice, typhus, cholera, smallpox, and diphtheria in studies to develop vaccines. Battle wounds were simulated, infected, and then randomly selected for sulfanilamide treatment or neglect. Persons were assigned to a study in which some drank desalinated water and others salt water until symptoms of iodine poisoning appeared. Various poisons were administered to observe the lethal effects. Men and women were sterilized in various ways to determine the most efficient methods for widespread population sterilization. The most notorious of the Nazi doctors, Josef Mengele, who escaped capture, was particularly interested in the genetic study of twins. He had collected twin children from the concentration camps, measured their physical features, performed cross-transfusions, transplanted genitals and other organs, and even created "artificial Siamese twins." He also used his twin collection for comparative drug studies, infecting one child and then killing both for study at autopsy.[4] Although most of the experiments were designed to solve urgent problems in military medicine, some research, particularly that of Dr. Mengele, was inspired by racist and pseudoscientific eugenics.

An American physician, Dr. Andrew C. Ivy, who had been chosen by the AMA to serve as the prosecution's medical expert, was largely responsible for the language of the Nuremberg Code. In preparatory notes for his court presentation, Dr. Ivy stated that "the rules of human experimentation had been well established by custom, social usage and the ethics of medical conduct." He then listed as the established rules all the provisions that appeared in the judges' version of the Code.[5]

The Nuremberg Doctors' Trial anticipated a major challenge to the long tradition of medical ethics. The Hippocratic *Oath* does not mention experimentation. Yet, the tradition had clearly proclaimed that no harm should be done to those who approach physicians for care. The *Oath* puts it more specifically: "no intentional harm or injustice." Physicians throughout history certainly did much harm with treatments that were ineffective and even destructive, but they were held never to *intend* harm: they must have the knowledge and skill to know how to avoid harm or how to balance any harm done with a benefit of health. It was not uncommon for medical men to assert that all treatments were experiments and, thus, that the physician is morally obliged to proceed with caution in all treatment. Scientific medicine, however, challenged that deontology. As it moved toward genuinely efficacious treatment, it would have to study that treatment by applying it to patients who might be harmed without promise of benefit. The atrocities of the Nazi doctors were brutal imitations of science, but true science itself had to advance by using human subjects. The ethics of experimentation with humans became the first serious challenge to the old tradition and brought into being the first agenda for the emerging bioethics.

April 25, 1953: DNA: The Secret of Life

On April 25, 1953, *Nature* published a one-page paper entitled "The Molecular Structure of Nucleic Acids" by James D. Watson and Francis H. Crick. The authors described the deoxyribonucleic acid (DNA) molecule, a fragment of matter hidden in the nucleus of almost all animal cells, as "two helical chains each coiled around the same axis."[6] The paper concluded, "It has not escaped our notice that the specific pairing we have postulated immediately suggests a possible copying mechanism for genetic material." The same fact did not escape the notice of many others. *The New York Times* promoted the authors' concluding remark to the headline of its report of the discovery: "Clue to Chemistry of Heredity Found."[7] The biochemical structure and function revealed by the Watson-Crick hypothesis, and by the torrent of scientific work that followed their observation, opens a wide realm of ethics with the words *genetic* and *heredity*. Those words cannot be uttered without raising perennial and profound human questions: What is it to be human? Is there a perfect form of humanity? If so, can it be achieved by human choice?

For almost a century, scientific interest in the mechanisms of heredity had been linked with political interest in the improvement of the human stock. A pseudoscience called *eugenics* appeared, claiming that its principles could discern between good and bad qualities for purposes of selecting better people to breed a better race. During the 1920s and 1930s in Great Britain, the home of eugenics, an intellectual debate ensued; in the United States, eugenicists went to work to classify human traits and enhance the national stock by enacting legal programs of sterilization and immigration restriction; in Germany eugenics was transformed into a monstrous policy of racial "cleansing." By the time Watson and Crick's paper was published, scientific genetics had divorced itself from eugenics, and eugenics itself was almost universally derided as bad science and contemptible politics. Still the implications of the new molecular biology for *genetic engineering* and *genetic control* awakened the ghost of eugenics. Racist and elitist visions reappeared, disguised as medical diagnosis and therapy. The means to turn those visions into reality were now more sophisticated than sterilization and abortion: they were the laboratory micromanipulations of the "secret of life." So, almost from the day Watson and Crick's paper was published, the ethics of the new genetics became a matter of concern to geneticists and to many others who were cognizant of the new science. The new genetics became the second topic on the agenda of the new bioethics.

December 23, 1954: Renal Transplantation

On December 23, 1954, Dr. Joseph E. Murray sutured a kidney excised from a 24-year-old man into his identical twin at the Peter Bent Brigham Hospital in Boston. The recipient not only survived during the critical days after the surgery while organ rejection threatened but lived for eight more years, eventually dying of coronary artery disease and glomerulonephritis.[8] Transplantation of tissue, limbs, and organs from one person to another had been a long desired but impossible dream. Yet, throughout the first half of the twentieth century, scientific and surgical progress had slowly brought the impossible dream toward reality.

Murray's bold surgery inaugurated the era of major organ transplantation. His experiment had succeeded due to the genetic similarity between the twins, a phenomenon that had been demonstrated some 20 years before by successful skin grafting between monzygotic twins. This genetic identity was a prerequisite for transplantation until drugs to counter immunological rejection were introduced in the 1960s, allowing transplantation from less than perfectly matched donors.[9]

Again the old imperative of medical ethics, "do no harm," was challenged. This maxim had always been understood to mean that any harm that might be done should contribute to the ultimate benefit of the patient. Excision of a healthy organ from a healthy donor was, under this interpretation, an impermissible harm. This medical maxim was taken for granted by jurisprudence, which would judge as a battery any intervention not intended to benefit the patient. Even the consent of the "battered" person did not justify the intervention. Other issues, such as the source and supply of organs, were equally troubling. The ethical and legal questions raised by this remarkable innovation—and its analogue, the use of artificial organs—entered the permanent agenda of the new medical ethics.

May 1960: Oral Contraceptives

In May 1960, the U.S. Food and Drug Administration approved Enovid, the first effective oral contraceptive. The "Pill," a combination of two synthetic steroids, progesterone and estrogen, was the product of basic biological research into the hormonal factors involved in conception, carried out with great creativity by

Dr. Gregory G. "Goody" Pincus and his group at the Worcester Foundation for Experimental Biology during the 1940s and 1950s. Their research was translated into pharmaceutical chemistry by the Searle Company. Initial clinical studies were planned and implemented during 1954–1955 by Dr. John Rock, Chairman of the Department of Obstetrics-Gynecology at Harvard. This laboratory and early clinical work was encouraged by the indefatigable crusader for birth control, Margaret Sanger. Large-scale clinical trials were inaugurated in Puerto Rico in April 1956. They demonstrated that Enovid was highly effective against pregnancy, with dizziness, headaches, and nausea as the only notable side effects.[10] Within three years, over 2 million American women were on the pill.

The pill posed, in new form, a very old ethical question: was it an unethical contravention of nature and God's law to prevent conception? That question was not, as some believe, an exclusive concern of the Roman Catholic Church: it had bothered Christian America throughout the nineteenth century. The advent of the pill raised the question again. For Catholics, it asked whether chemical contraception was morally equivalent to physical contraception. For the general public, which had widely accepted contraception as moral and as a great benefit for women, the question was whether the ready availability of an effective, easy contraceptive would revolutionize the social and sexual life of Americans.

March 9, 1960: Chronic Hemodialysis and the Seattle Dialysis Selection Committee

In Seattle, Washington, on March 9, 1960, a small loop of plastic was sutured into a vein and an artery in the forearm of Clyde Shields, a 39-year-old machinist dying of renal failure. This plastic arteriovenous shunt and cannula allowed Mr. Shields to be connected to a hemodialysis machine, which cleansed his blood of metabolically accumulated poisons that his diseased kidneys could not eliminate. The shunt had been invented a month earlier by Dr. Belding H. Scribner, a nephrologist on the faculty of the University of Washington School of Medicine, with the aid of a biomedical engineer, William Quentin. The dialysis machine itself had been in use since its invention by Dr. Willem Kolff in the Nazi-occupied Netherlands. Although the dialysis machine worked well for persons afflicted with acute kidney failure due to trauma or poisoning, whose blood could be cleansed in a few treatments, it could not be used for patients with chronic kidney failure because the required surgical hookup could be performed only several times. Dr. Scribner's invention made chronic dialysis possible: patients could be hooked up and unhooked with ease, sustaining their lives for indefinite periods and, even better, returning them to active daily life.

The success of chronic dialysis treatment created a practical problem. The original Seattle Artificial Kidney Center had a nine-bed capacity; dialysis was a rarified medical treatment, not easily initiated in many places. It was estimated that about 20,000 people annually in the United States suffered from end-stage renal disease. Persons who begin dialysis do not die but live in continual dependence on the machine. New patients constantly arrive. How could the capacity be expanded to meet this never-ending need? Also, the treatment was very expensive; patients had to pay about $10,000 annually in 1960 dollars, a daunting sum for many patients, even those with insurance, whose insurance companies hesitated to pay for experimental treatment.

The Seattle Artificial Kidney Center took an unprecedented approach to this unique problem of resource allocation. An Admissions and Policy Committee was formed to select, from the group of patients considered by physicians as medically and psychiatrically suitable for this rigorous treatment, those few who would be offered dialysis. The committee was composed of seven members with varied backgrounds: a minister, a lawyer, a homemaker, a businessman, a labor leader, and two physicians from specialties other than renal medicine. The anonymity of the members was protected. Rather than creating abstract criteria for selection, the committee members began to work case by case, reviewing extensive personal, social, psychological, and economic information on the candidates, none of whom they knew by name or in person. Gradually they drew up a list of considerations that they judged relevant: age, gender, marital status and number of dependants, income, educational background, occupation, past performance, and future potential. For the next four years, the committee used these rough criteria, which came to be designated *social worth criteria*, to perform their agonizing task of choosing "who shall live and who shall die."

Despite its efforts at anonymity, the committee was a magnet for media coverage, and its activity became the object of criticism by scholars.[11] One article described the committee's deliberations as "polluted by prejudices and mindless clichés" and warned that "the Seattle committee measured persons in accord with its own middle-class suburban values . . . this rules out the creative nonconformists, who rub the bourgeoisie the wrong way but who historically have contributed much to the making of America. The Pacific Northwest is no place for a Henry David Thoreau with bad kidneys."[12] Philosophers and theologians made meticulous analyses of the values and principles involved in selecting persons for scarce lifesaving technologies.[13]

The Seattle dialysis program, with its unusual selection process, was a dramatic instance of the new medicine meeting traditional medical ethics: one of the first genuinely life-sustaining therapies that challenged the loyalty of the physician to the single patient for whom he or she is caring. The idea of turning over this responsibility to a lay committee was shocking. The idea of choosing patients for life or for death, although familiar to medicine in emergency triage, seemed appalling when it came to the common use of a lifesaving treatment. The morality of patients' removing themselves from a life-sustaining machine reminded some of suicide. The problem of selecting patients for dialysis was generalizable to the whole field of transplantation and the use of other scarce resources. The public attention that this event aroused, and the scholarly debate that it stimulated were unprecedented.

December 3, 1967: Heart Transplantation

The transplantation story, which had begun with Dr. Joseph Murray's success in transplanting kidneys, came to a stunning climax on December 3, 1967. Dr. Christiaan Barnard of the Groote Schur Hospital in Cape Town, South Africa, took a beating heart from Denise Darvall, who had been admitted with "irreversibly fatal brain damage" due to a vehicular accident, and placed it in the chest of 55-year-old Louis Washkansky, who was in critical cardiac failure. Washkansky died 18 days after the operation. *Time* magazine hailed this feat as "the ultimate operation," and media coverage worldwide was intense.[14]

The South African surgeon was not discouraged by Washkansky's death. Only a few weeks later, he transplanted the heart of Clive Haupt into Dentist Philip Blaiberg, who lived for 594 days. The following year, over 100 heart transplants were performed around the world. The results were discouraging. By August 1969, only 37 of 142 patients transplanted during the previous 20 months were alive; in June 1970, 10 survivors were counted among 160 transplant recipients. Transplant surgeons themselves slowed their pace, returning to the laboratory to find more effective defenses against immunological rejection.

However, the new form of transplantation pushed to the fore another unprecedented ethical problem: the determination of death of those whose hearts were to be taken for transplantation. Renal transplantation also raised the question, since cadaver donors were an alternative, though a less desirable, source of organs. Unlike renal transplantation, in which one kidney can be taken safely from a living and consenting donor, heart transplants must always come from one whose death is associated with the taking of the organ. Traditionally, law and ethics had determined that death occurred when the heart stopped beating and breathing ceased. Now, continued circulation was necessary to preserve a viable organ for transplant. Thus, the problem of defining death in terms other than cessation of cardiac and respiratory function became a pressing matter.[15]

August 5, 1968: Harvard Definition of Brain Death

A step toward the solution of this dilemma appeared in *The New England Journal of Medicine* on August 5, 1968. "A Definition of Irreversible Coma: Report of the Ad Hoc Committee at Harvard Medical School to Examine the Definition of

Brain Death" began: "Our primary purpose is to define irreversible coma as a new criterion for death." The report explains why: "improvements in resuscitative and supportive measures have led to increased efforts to save those who are desperately injured." Partial success at resuscitation leaves living persons whose brains are irreversibly damaged, inflicting terrible burdens on themselves and their families. A second reason is that "obsolete criteria for the definition of death can lead to controversy in obtaining organs for transplantation." In light of these purposes, the ad hoc committee concluded that "responsible medical opinion is now ready to adopt new criteria for pronouncing death to have occurred in an individual sustaining irreversible coma as a result of permanent brain damage."[16]

The problem that the ad hoc committee wished to address had its root in the "obsolete . . . definition of death." For centuries, doctors had recognized that death occurred when a person's breathing and pulse ceased, and the law had required that doctors declare death when they were assured of "an irreversible cessation of respiration and circulation." The modern respirator, however, could support breathing even when consciousness had been irretrievably lost. Also, the exigencies of heart transplantation created a paradox. A heart could not be taken from a living, that is, breathing, person, since removal of the heart would cause death. At the same time, if the heart remained even for a short time in a body no longer breathing, the physiological properties that made it useful as a transplant deteriorated. As transplantation from cadavers became more common, confusion reigned. Papers in the medical literature demonstrated uncertainty: persons who were the sources of organs were described as "dead" or "immanently dead" or "irreversibly dying." Problematic legal cases had already arisen.[17]

The Harvard Report presents these complex issues in a three-page article. It describes the physical and neurological characteristics of *irreversible coma*: unresponsiveness, no movements or breathing, no reflexes, and a flat electroencephalogram indicating a state of permanent and irreversible coma. That description is followed by a legal commentary that explains the inadequacy of the obsolete definition, namely, the absence of all vital signs. Finally, a brief section cites the words of Pope Pius XII endorsing the venerable doctrine that "extraordinary means" need not be used to sustain life. The Report's only citation is to the papal statement.[18]

Response to the Harvard Report was swift. In 1970, Kansas enacted legislation that recognized the "new criterion," allowing "absence of spontaneous brain function" to serve alongside "absence of spontaneous respiration and circulation" as a definition of death.[19] Many states followed suit, but with widely differing statutory language. It was possible to be dead one way in one state and dead in another way in a neighboring state. The confusion that the Harvard ad hoc committee had hoped to dispel returned and provided bioethics with another question.

July 26, 1972: The Tuskegee Revelations

On July 26, 1972, *The New York Times* announced, "For forty years, the United States Public Health Service has conducted a study in which human beings with syphilis, who were induced to serve as guinea pigs, have gone without treatment for the disease . . . the study was conducted to determine from autopsies what the disease does to the human body." The subjects of the study were "about 600 black men, mostly poor and uneducated, from Tuskegee, Alabama." The men had been promised "free transportation to and from hospitals, free hot lunches, free medical care for any disease other than syphilis and free burial after autopsies were performed."[20] In the following days and weeks, details of the Tuskegee Study were revealed in the press. Of the 600 research subjects, 400 had diagnosed syphilis but were never told and never treated. They were never informed that they were research subjects or that treatment for their condition could have been provided. The other 200, who did not have syphilis, were controls. All of these men, patients and controls alike, were told that they had "bad blood" and were informed that they required periodic medical examinations, including spinal taps. When the story broke in 1972, 74 of the untreated subjects were still living.

The syphilis study had begun in 1932 after a Public Health Service Venereal Disease Treatment program, initiated several years before in Macon County, Alabama, lost its funding. It occurred to the Public Health Service officer in charge of the treatment program, Dr. Taliaferro Clark, that the population of Macon County, which had one of the highest rates of syphilis in the country, offered an unparalleled opportunity to study the natural history of syphilis in the untreated patient. At that time, the standard treatment with arsenical and mercurial medications was arduous and of dubious efficacy. The collaboration of the hospital at one of the nation's premier African-American educational establishments, Tuskegee Institute, was secured. The study, initially planned for 1 year, persisted for 40 years, even after effective treatment with penicillin became available. On a number of occasions, officials of the Public Health Service had evaluated the study and decided that its scientific value justified its continuance.

On August 24, 1972, the Department of Health, Education and Welfare appointed the Tuskegee Syphilis Study Ad Hoc Panel, consisting of nine persons, to determine whether the Tuskegee Study was justified at its beginning and after penicillin became available; to recommend whether it should be continued, or, if not, how it should be terminated "in a way consistent with the rights and health needs of its remaining participants"; and to determine whether the rights of patients participating in research sponsored by the Department of Health, Education and Welfare were adequately protected. The panel's final report, issued on April 28, 1973, concluded that the study was unethical in its beginnings, criticized the failure to terminate the study when effective therapy appeared, and recommended strict oversight of medical research.[21]

Several other events during the second half of the 1960s cast suspicion on the probity of scientific researchers. Doctors from the Sloan-Kettering Cancer Center in New York City had received authorization from the administrators of the Jewish Chronic Disease Hospital in Brooklyn to implant cancer cells under the skin of aged, debilitated patients without their knowledge or consent. Researchers from New York University School of Medicine had been authorized by administrators of New York State's Willowbrook Hospital to infect retarded children with the hepatitis virus. Both of these events, when publicized in the media, shocked the public, but no event had more impact on the public conscience than the Tuskegee Study. Its revelation appeared at a time of heightened concern and anger about racial discrimination and heightened sensitivity to the abuse of the poor and powerless. The revelations seemed to bring the horrors of the Nazi medical experiments, which many had judged impossible in the United States, into our benign scientific and medical world. The ethics of research, which had been under quiet scrutiny for a decade, burst forth into public view.

January 22, 1973: Roe v. Wade

On January 22, 1973, the U.S. Supreme Court announced its decision in *Roe v. Wade*, a case brought by a Texas woman against the District Attorney of Dallas County. She charged that the state's criminal abortion statute, dating from the nineteenth century, which exempted from criminality only an abortion performed to save the mother's life, prevented her from obtaining a desired abortion. The Court's decision held that state law could not restrict the right of a woman, in accord with her doctor, to obtain an abortion during the first trimester of pregnancy. It further held that states could make laws regulating the safety of abortion procedures relative to maternal health during the second trimester and that during the third trimester, when the fetus was "viable," law could prohibit abortion except when necessary to preserve the life and health of the woman. The Court justified these holdings by asserting that the U.S. Constitution contains an implicit right to privacy, implied by several explicit provisions of the Bill of Rights. The Court also affirmed that a fetus is not a person, as interpreted under the 14th Amendment to the Constitution, and thus does not have the rights guaranteed by the Constitution. The decision noted, "we need not resolve the difficult question of when life begins. When those trained in the respective disciplines of medicine, philosophy and theology are unable to arrive at any consensus, the judiciary, at this point in the development of man's knowledge, is not in a position to speculate as to the answer." Nevertheless, the Court allowed that the medical determination of viability, "the capability of meaningful life outside the womb," could be a "compelling point" at which a state might legitimately protect fetal life.[22]

Roe v. Wade came after a century and a half of restrictive abortion law in the United States. The Court's decision was a radical reform of American law, but it appeared, at the time, to be consistent with a more liberal attitude of Americans toward abortion. This appearance proved deceptive. As state after state revised their old statutes to conform with the Supreme Court's ruling, millions of citizens slowly began to express their dissent. By the mid-1970s, abortion had become a major political issue with deep moral implications.[23] At the same time, the profound question of when life begins, most obvious in abortion, attended the rapidly advancing field of reproductive technology. It became a central question for the new bioethics.

April 14, 1975: Karen Ann Quinlan

On April 14, 1975, 21-year-old Karen Ann Quinlan was brought to the emergency department of Newton Memorial Hospital in Newton, New Jersey. She was comatose. Her coma had resulted, it appeared, from ingestion of barbiturates, Valium, and alcohol. She was put on a respirator to assist her breathing. She was soon transferred to a major medical center where, over the next five months, her neurological condition deteriorated. Neurologists stated that she was in a *persistent vegetative state*, the technical name for her neurological condition: she had lost all consciousness and was unlikely ever to regain it, although her vegetative functions—respiration, circulation, nutrition, and elimination—might continue indefinitely. Her parents, Mr. and Mrs. Joseph Quinlan, had decided, after much prayerful agony and consultation, to request the doctors to remove Karen's breathing tube and allow her to die. The attending physician, Dr. Robert Morse, after consulting the hospital's lawyer and ascertaining that discontinuing life support might lead to criminal charges, declined to disconnect Karen's respirator. Mr. Quinlan petitioned the court for an injunction requiring the hospital to stop providing medical treatment to Karen.

The case reached the New Jersey Supreme Court. On March 31, 1976, the justices concluded that, under the protection of an implicit privacy right granted by the Constitution, Karen Ann, "if miraculously lucid for an interval . . . and perceptive of her irreversible condition, could effectively decide upon discontinuance of the life-support apparatus even if it meant the prospect of natural death" and that Karen's parents were appropriate surrogates to exercise that right for her. The state, said the justices, has no compelling interest in forcing Karen "to endure the unendurable, only to vegetate a few measurable months with no realistic possibility of returning to any semblance of cognitive or sapient life."[24] There would be no civil or criminal liability should life support be discontinued. The New Jersey judgment granted relief to Karen Ann Quinlan. Her father again ordered the discontinuance of the respirator; physicians began to wean her from the machine and removed her totally from it on May 20. Unexpectedly, she began to breath spontaneously. On June 9, she was moved from St. Claire's Hospital to a nursing home, where she lived in a persistent vegetative state for 10 years, dying on June 11, 1985, at the age of 31.

Karen Ann's story, covered assiduously by the media, had made the American public more aware of the tragic side of the miracle of intensive care. American law began to move toward views that could accommodate the undesirable consequences of technological medicine. American doctors began to attend more seriously to the ethical dimensions of clinical decisions to withhold or withdraw life-sustaining treatment. Bioethics inherited the task of delineating the principles and values that would shape those ethical dimensions.

July 25, 1978: Baby Louise Brown

On July 25, 1978, Louise Joy Brown was born near Manchester, England. Her parents, John and Leslie Brown, an English working-class couple, had reason to call their baby Joy. After nine years of trying to become pregnant, Mrs. Brown had been told that her fallopian tubes had been damaged by an earlier ectopic pregnancy and that she would not be able to conceive. The Browns were referred to Patrick C. Steptoe, an obstetrician who had been collaborating with Cambridge physiologist Robert G. Edwards on perfecting the conditions for retrieval of oocytes, fertilization of the retrieved oocytes under laboratory conditions (in vitro), and implantation of the fertilized embryo in the womb. Mrs. Brown was the first of their experimental subjects to carry her implanted embryo to term. On the morning after Louise's birth, media around the world proclaimed the birth of the world's first "test tube baby."

Professor Edwards and Mr. Steptoe, with the cooperation of Mr. and Mrs. Brown, had achieved a long-sought goal: a technical remedy for female infertility. That procedure could bring the joy of a child to couples whose infertility was due to physical constrictures of the fallopian tubes. As the scientist and obstetrician offered that remedy, they stirred an ethical maelstrom. Not only did their technique offer a solution for the personal tragedy of infertility, it also placed within reach the human conceptus, opening possibilities for manipulating, designing, and cloning human beings. It also raised two questions. Was it ethical to create babies in a petri dish rather than within a mother's body? Should the fashioning of humans according to deliberate design ever be allowed? Issues about ownership of fertilized embryos, rightful claims of parenthood among the multiple contributors to a child's being, and preimplantation research and diagnosis pressed on public policy and the law. Each of those questions provided ample material for the reflections of bioethicists.[25]

Spring, 1982: Baby Doe

Since the 1970s, the new medical specialty of neonatology, dedicated to saving the lives of premature infants, had struggled with a moral dilemma: should all newborn babies be rescued from death, even if their prospects for life or for normal life were very dismal? In 1973, an article by Drs. Raymond Duff and Alastair Campbell, "Moral and Ethical Dilemmas in the Special-Care Nursery," revealed to the world what neonatologists understood only too well: many of the tiny premature babies who needed the technology of the intensive-care nursery failed to respond to the therapeutic rigors of that technology and were allowed to die by being deliberately removed from the ventilators.[26] Until that article was published and reported in the media, few had known how anguishing a drama of life and death was being played in the isolettes of the intensive-care nursery.

That drama moved to the stage of public policy in 1982. In April of that year, a baby with Down's syndrome and a blocked intestine was born in Bloomington, Indiana. Surgeons could easily correct the blocked bowel, but the baby's developmental disability was permanent. The child's parents declined permission for surgery to correct the intestinal defect, preferring to see their baby die rather than grow up mentally retarded. The hospital sought a court order to perform the surgery over the parents' objections. After the Indiana courts upheld the parents' decision, the case was reported in the press and on television, and the baby, who had died on April 15, christened only with the legal name Baby Doe, became famous.[27] It is said that President Ronald Reagan saw the television report and immediately ordered his Secretary of Health and Human Services, Richard Schweiker, to ensure that this decision would be prevented in the future. "The President," said Secretary Schweiker, "has instructed me to make absolutely clear to health providers in this nation that Federal law does not allow medical discrimination against handicapped infants."[28]

In response to President Reagan's request, Secretary Schweiker issued regulations in March 1983, requiring that intensive-care nurseries and maternity wards display notices stating that "Discriminatory failure to feed and care for handicapped infants in this facility is prohibited by Federal law."[29] The notices carried a toll-free Handicapped Infant Hotline telephone number where suspected violations could be reported to a Department of Health and Human Services (DHHS) "Baby Doe Squad" for investigation. The American Academy of Pediatrics immediately challenged these regulations. A complicated legal battle followed, taking Baby Doe's story to the U.S. Supreme Court, which invalidated the regulations of the DHHS. Justice John Paul Stevens wrote, "the Federal Government has no power to overrule parental decisions . . . the Administration had presented no evidence that would justify Federal intervention in an area traditionally controlled by the state."[30]

Some members of Congress were determined to find a judge-proof way to protect babies from what they saw as a form of medical murder akin to abortion. They succeeded in passing Public Law 98-457, signed into law by President Reagan on October 9, 1984. On the third anniversary of Baby Doe's death, April 15, 1985, the DHHS issued regulations and interpretive guidelines to implement the new federal law. The regulations required that all medically indicated treatments be provided to infants unless "such treatment would merely prolong dying, not be effective in ameliorating or correcting all of the infant's life-threatening conditions, or otherwise be futile in terms of the survival of the infant."[31] States were required to carry out surveillance of neonatal intensive-care units for violations of the rules or lose federal funding for their child protective services. The ethics of neonatal intensive care was added to the issues that would generate a new ethics of medicine.

December 3, 1982: The Artificial Heart

Seattle dentist Dr. Barney Clark, age 61, was a very sick man, suffering from chronic obstructive pulmonary disease, emphysema, and cardiomyopathy. He had smoked heavily from his 20s until he turned 50, but his lung and heart problems worsened, forcing him to retire from practice at age 55. His desperate condition and his age disqualified him from heart transplantation programs. He then learned that a surgeon at the University of Utah, Dr. William C. DeVries, was seeking an appropriate candidate for the first implantation of a mechanical heart devised by his colleague, Robert Jarvik. Clark's diagnosis of idiopathic cardiomyopathy with Class IV congestive failure met DeVries' requirements, and Clark agreed to be his first patient. Just before midnight on December 1, 1982, his fleshy heart was replaced by a device of plastic and fabric, connected by a thick hose through his chest to a pneumatic pump by his bedside. Clark's postoperative course was difficult: air leaks in the chest, blood clots, seizures, a ruptured valve on the mechanical heart, and only intermittent lucidity made the next few weeks a horror. He improved briefly and was being prepared for transfer to an extended-care facility, when his condition worsened. On March 23, 1983, Barney Clark died of circulatory collapse due to multiorgan system failure.

During those 112 days of life on a mechanical heart, Barney Clark became a media celebrity. Reporters settled in at the hospital, and the hospital's regular releases on Clark's condition became the stuff of headlines and the nightly news. Clark's survival, miserable though it was, encouraged doctors enough to attempt implants on a dozen more patients, but with little success. The profession again called an informal moratorium on artificial heart implantation, but the sad episodes gave bioethics another example of the problem of technology: what should count as a benefit, who should decide how to use it, and who should pay for its costs?[32]

April 11, 1983: The AIDS Epidemic

The AIDS epidemic did not begin on April 11, 1983: it was at least two years old on that date. However, on April 11, two events coincided to dramatize it. *Newsweek* magazine, published on that day, splashed the word *epidemic* across its cover: "EPIDEMIC: The Mysterious and Deadly Disease Called AIDS May Be the Public Health Threat of the Century. How Did It Start? How Can It Be Stopped?" On the same day, Dr. Robert Gallo, a National Institutes of Health scientist, announced to the first National Cancer Institute conference on AIDS that he suspected a retrovirus to be the cause of the syndrome. Randy Shilts, historian of the epidemic, says of that issue of *Newsweek*, "with AIDS finally ensconced as a legitimate news story, an avalanche of coverage began." And Gallo's announcement, Shilts writes, "was later cited by the officials of the National Cancer Institute as the turning point, the time that the Institute became firmly committed to finding the cause of AIDS."[33]

    In 1981, physicians around the country had begun to see unusual complexes of symptoms in young male patients: fatigue, fever, wasting, swollen lymph nodes, incessant respiratory and other infections, and uncommon skin cancers. Some mysterious impairment of the immune system and an unknown infectious agent were suspected causes of this disease, which proved inevitably fatal in a short time. Often, the patients with these perplexing symptoms were gay men. In 1982 physicians had constructed a clinical diagnosis to which the ugly acronym *GRID* (*gay-related immunodeficiency*) was applied. As reports filtered into the Centers for Disease Control (CDC) in Atlanta, it became apparent that persons other than gay men were also affected. Persons who had received blood transfusions or regularly used blood products for treatment of hemophilia were among the affected. The label *GRID*, clearly no longer appropriate, was discarded in favor of *AIDS* (*acquired immune deficiency syndrome*). As a clearer clinical picture of AIDS emerged, the gay community started to realize that it was being decimated by a lethal epidemic; public health officials became concerned and slowly began to organize a response; and the public learned, in fragmented and often distorted ways, that there was a new plague in the land. By April 1983, 1295 Americans had contracted AIDS; 492 had died, and unknown thousands more harbored the lethal virus. Never before had the traditional strategies for epidemic control been implemented under constraints such as consent and confidentiality; never before had the awareness of discrimination and stigma, the inevitable familiars of epidemic disease, been so heightened.[34]

9

Conclusion
From Medical Ethics to Bioethics

The chronicle of ethical events opened with the Nuremberg Doctors' Trial, whose defendants had committed a moral outrage against the long tradition of medicine's duty to protect the sick. It ended with the story of moral perplexity about how to protect the sick in the midst of a disease that threatens society. During the years covered by the chronicle, medical science and medical practice had changed dramatically. New techniques, from antibiotics to transplanted and artificial organs, genetic discoveries, and reproductive manipulations, together with the research that engendered them, presented the public, scientists, doctors, and politicians with questions that had never before been asked. Answers were needed for personal choices and for policy decisions. These events took place in a cultural and a social environment that fostered those questions. During the 1960s, the United States had entered a period of anguished introspection about its own moral ideals as the Vietnam War eroded confidence in the probity of government and the honor of the military, and as the civil rights movement aroused moral anger and shame. These moral questions spilled over into the apparently benign world of medicine and health care. In particular, the revelation of the Tuskegee experiments, which linked medical progress with racial discrimination, shocked the nation.

Many scientists, whose consciences had been troubled by the destructive effects of the marvelous harnessing of nuclear power, began to wonder about the ambiguity of advances in medical science. Discussions of these ambiguities were arranged at many scientific conferences during the 1950s and 1960s. Gradually, scholars from the two academic disciplines that had traditionally studied morality, philosophy and theology, began to join the scientists. Their appearance at these events drew the wide-ranging discussions into more articulate and organized expositions. Two research centers were founded in 1969 and 1971, the Institute of Ethics, Society and the Life Sciences (now known as the Hastings Center) and the Kennedy Institute of Ethics at Georgetown University. From the Hastings

Center came a steady stream of carefully considered opinions, worked out by small groups of scholars from different disciplines called together to discuss specific issues in detail. From the Kennedy Institute came a four-volume *Encyclopedia of Bioethics* (1975) and the annual publication of the *Bibliography of Bioethics*, which, in volumes of steadily increasing size, registered the growing literature in the field.

Just at that time, Paul Ramsey and Hans Jonas, leading figures in their respective fields of theology and philosophy, wrote articulate analyses of particular problems facing scientists and physicians. Jonas produced essays on the ethics of research with humans and on the definition of death; Ramsey published a book, *Patient as Person*, that cast an acute, critical light on such questions as informed consent, organ transplantation, and research with children.[1] Their work made it evident that the concepts and methods of the classical disciplines that studied the moral life could be usefully and carefully applied to the new problems. Philosophers, theologians, lawyers, and sociologists who created that literature found themselves migrating out of their original disciplines into a new field of scholarly endeavor. Many found themselves employed as professors of bioethics in the nation's schools of medicine, called upon not only to teach medical students but also to address medical audiences, consult with clinicians, participate in professional committees and councils, and appear before governmental inquiries. Professors, as is their way, created curricula, wrote textbooks, and explored theoretical concepts that might draw the classical disciplines dealing with morality, into closer contact with the practical questions about the pursuit of science and the practice of medicine. The word *bioethics* had been invented in the late 1960s to designate a vision of a world in which scientific advances were linked to human and environmental values in an evolutionary progress toward human community. By the end of the 1970s, bioethics described more than a vision: it designated a new discipline with a distinctive literature and all the panoply of courses and conferences that academic disciplines engender.[2]

The bioethicists brought to this discourse concepts and methods that had been honed in their original disciplines but had rarely been used in the long tradition of medical decorum, deontology, and politic ethics. Concepts such as *autonomy* and *justice* entered the vocabulary of medical ethics; old maxims such as those about "ordinary and extraordinary means of care" and "double effect" were subjected to critical refurbishing, and assumptions about the physician's authority, the right to experiment, and euthanasia were rigorously examined. Perhaps the most dramatic innovation was the insertion of the concept of respect for the autonomy of the patient into the heart of the ethics of medicine. The long tradition had, almost without exception, revered the concept of benign paternalism, the duty of the physician to determine the best course for the patient according to his ability and judgment. The new concerns about medical technology, combined with a growing skepticism in all areas of life about the impartiality of professional experts, summoned a principle unfamiliar to traditional medical ethics but familiar to philosophers: the freedom of persons to judge what is in their benefit without interference from others. In light of this principle, many elements of the old ethics, such as telling the truth to patients, experimenting on their bodies, and choosing to accept or refuse a course of treatment, were drastically reformulated.

In the United States, one event more than any other propelled the old medical ethics into the world of bioethics. After the revelations of the Tuskegee Syphilis Study and several other instances of questionably ethical research, the U.S. Congress, which funded most of this research with grants from the National Institutes of Health, established the National Commission for the Protection of Human Subjects of Biomedical and Behavioral Research. The task of this Commission, which sat from 1974 to 1978, was to recommend to the federal government regulations that would protect the rights and welfare of human research subjects and to develop the moral principles that should underlie such research. As it worked on these issues, the Commission summoned many scholars from a variety of disciplines, inviting them to present their views in testimony and in extended essays on the nature of the ethical questions. A substantial body of thoughtful analysis was produced in which notions were defined and arguments articulated. Many scholars who had never before ruminated about the ethical issues facing science and medicine were recruited into the intellectual dialogue. After the National Commission completed its work, Congress established a successsor, the President's Commission for the Study of Ethical Problems in Medicine and Biomedical and Behavioral Research. That Commission delved into the issues surrounding life-sustaining treatment, the definition of death, screening and testing for genetic disease, and genetic engineering. Again the Commission's deliberations drew on the advice of many scholars and practitioners, as well as the opinions of the broader public. Its reports gave solid evidence that the bioethics that had begun as a catalogue of questions had evolved into a discipline of respectable scholarship and widespread public influence.[3]

Even the shrine of traditional medical ethics, the American Medical Association, was reconstructed. Although the 1847 Code of Ethics had been revised five times (1903, 1912, 1947, 1957, and 1980), it remained a compendium of the traditional deontology, decorum, and politic ethics, compressed over time from 48 sections to 7 sentences. However, in 1985, the body charged with interpretation of the *Principles* had its name changed from Judicial Council to Council on Ethical and Judicial Affairs. Its role was expanded from guardian of the *Principles* to investigator and advisor on many of the new issues. Over the last decade, it has issued opinions on the ethical problems raised by reproductive technology, genetics, organ transplantation, care of the dying, and euthanasia, and the treatment of persons with human immunodeficiency virus infection, as well as on the more traditional questions about confidentiality, consultation, conflict of interest, and medical discipline. These opinions have been informed by the scholarly studies that were appearing in the bioethical literature.[4] Other major health care organizations created ethics committees and issued statements of a similar nature on the ethical problems associated with their specialties.

During the 1970s and 1980s, scholars, commissions and committees worked hard on the concepts and arguments surrounding these issues. In so doing, they not only clarified the issues themselves, but also improved their own understanding of how to analyze and argue about bioethical questions. Many scholars who had previously known of these issues only as observers, if at all, were attracted to their study. They became the original bioethicists. Many of them were appointed to medical school faculties as full time professors of bioethics. In addition to these scholars, many other persons, both professional and lay, became peripherally involved in bioethics. Government regulations about research with human subjects required all research institutions to have an Institutional Review Board (IRB) charged with review and approval of all scientific proposals in which human subjects were involved. Hundreds of these IRBs came into being, and thousands of physicians, scientists, and others became familiar with the principles of ethical research, the regulations to protect the subjects' welfare and rights, and their application to particular cases. Similarly, in the late 1970s, hospitals began to establish ethics committees to deal with the complex problems of deciding when life support should be discontinued for particular patients. These committees, which were advisory to physicians and to the institution, undertook to clarify policies about resuscitation and life support. Again, many persons who served on these committees became familiar with the language, concepts, and literature of bioethics. Around the country, conferences and courses were held, and books and journals appeared for this new population of part-time bioethicists.

The discipline of bioethics is not unified by a single dominant theory or methodology. It reflects the circumstances of its evolution: questions about the ethical dimensions of science and medicine were raised and debated by a variety of commentators, scientists and physicians, lawyers, politicians and public policy experts, social scientists, philosophers, and theologians. These highly interdisciplinary discussions brought considerations from every side into the debate. The two disciplines most familiar with the logic and rhetoric of ethics, moral philosophy and moral theology, provided their skills for the debates and, in so doing, often transformed the desultory discussion common to ethical discourse into formats with distinct definitions and logical arguments. They did not, however, submerge the interdisciplinary features in any single ethical theory. Even though some bioethicists have attempted to formulate overarching theories, the discipline welcomes a wide range of arguments, views, and methods. Those familiar with moral philosophy might notice a preponderance of *rule utilitarianism* in the products of bioethical reflections: moral questions are argued in terms of some rather consistent moral rules, such as "do no harm," and those rules are justified by reference to a general conception of personal and social welfare. One rule in particular, respect for the autonomy of persons, holds a particularly important, almost absolute, place in this rule utilitarianism. But even this powerful rule does not dominate, excluding other rules about beneficence and justice, nor does it crush the relevance of circumstances of cases. Because bioethics has a practical end, to guide decisions and to shape policy, it is not rare that out of the welter of argument comes substantial consensus.[5]

In the quarter century since the discipline of bioethics was born, it has established itself as an integral branch of practical or applied philosophy and as a valuable adjunct to health policy and medical practice. It has developed some methodologies for dealing with the questions to which it is devoted. Those questions touch the human condition so deeply that no final answers will ever be given, but continued examination remains necessary and tentative recommendations must be offered. New questions arise as new technical possibilities emerge from science and as new social arrangements appear. Bioethics today is much better prepared intellectually to study these questions than it was in its infancy. Its task is to promote clarity in the debates and to criticize simple solutions to complex issues.

Parallel developments took place around the world. Interest in the ethical dilemmas of the new medicine appeared in Great Britain almost contemporaneously with the United States. In Europe, concern about ethical medicine was compelled by the Nazi outrages: experimentation with human subjects, euthanasia, and the use of genetics for "ethnic cleansing" had tainted medicine. On the Asian and Latin American continents, the rapid advances in technological medicine in poor countries raised questions about allocation of resources. In all these places, educational institutions, professional associations, and political bodies turned their attention to the ethics of the new medicine and found that the traditions of their cultures were only partially prepared to meet the challenges.

The history of ethics in medicine is long and complex. This book has tried to show that, in literate medicine everywhere, certain themes of deontology, decorum, and politic ethics appear. Although these themes are culturally varied, they show similarities, much as a human kinship originates in "the old country" and then emigrates to several new lands. The long tradition of medical ethics has preserved those themes over the centuries. Only recently, however, has a new theme emerged, one worthy of a new name, bioethics. That new theme welcomes, more than ever before, a careful and deep examination of the moral dilemmas of medicine. It welcomes into the discussion persons from outside medicine and incorporates the results of deliberations by councils, committees, and commissions that often included as many laypersons as professionals. It even welcomes into the heart of the long tradition novel values and principles, and allows them to revise the institutions in which medicine is practiced. Historian David Rothman writes,

"By 1978 . . . bioethics was a field, would-be ethicists had career lines to follow and the notion that medical ethics belonged exclusively to medicine had been forgotten by almost everyone, except for a cadre of older physicians and a handful of historians. . . . The record, I believe, makes a convincing case for a fundamental transformation in the style as well as the substance of medical decision making."[6]

Notes

Preface

1. Andrew Wear, Johanna Geyer-Kordesch, and Roger French (eds.), *Doctors and Ethics: The Earlier Historical Setting of Professional Ethics* (Amsterdam: Rodopi, 1993). This collection of essays, together with Robert Baker, Dorothy Porter, and Roy Porter (eds.), *The Codification of Medical Morality in the Eighteenth and Nineteenth Century* (Dordrecht/ Boston: Kluwer Academic Publishers, 1993), both produced by scholars associated with London's Wellcome Institute for the History of Medicine, start to fill the gap; this history is much indebted to their contents. Chester Burns (ed.), *Legacies in Ethics and Medicine* (New York: Science History Publications, 1977), collected 16 articles on the history of medical ethics that had appeared before 1977. The entry "Medical ethics, history of" in Warren Reich (ed.) *Encyclopedia of Bioethics* (New York: Simon and Shuster, 1995) contains many fine articles. Robert Baker and Laurence McCullough are planning *The Cambridge History of Medical Ethics* as a compendious review of the subject. It is expected to be published in 2002. Any history of medical ethics must be read against the background of the general history of medicine. The most recent of the many general histories is Roy Porter, *The Greatest Benefit to Mankind. A Medical History of Mankind* (New York: W.W. Norton, 1997). A reader of the history of medical *ethics* might benefit from the history of ethics: see Alasdair MacIntyre, *A Short History of Ethics* (New York: Macmillan, 1966). The same author warns about the dangers of transporting moral notions from one culture into another in his *After Virtue* (Notre Dame: University of Notre Dame Press, 1984).

Introduction: The Long Tradition of Ethics in Medicine

1. The phrase *the long tradition* is borrowed from Mary Catherine Welborn, "The long tradition: a study in fourteenth-century medical deontology," in James L. Cate and Eugene N. Anderson (eds.), *Medieval and Historiographical Essays in Honor of James Westfall Thompson* (Chicago: University of Chicago Press, 1938). Criticism of the long tradition concept is found in Robert M. Veatch and Carol G. Mason, "Hippocratic vs. Judeo-Christian medical ethics: principles in conflict," *Journal of Religious Ethics* 15 (1986): 86–105.

2. Aristotle, *Ethics* I, ii, 1094a22, trans. H. Rackham (Cambridge: Harvard University Press, 1926), p. 5.

3. Eliot Friedson, *Doctoring Together: A Study of Professional Social Control* (New York: Elsevier, 1975), p. 245.

1. Hellenic, Hellenistic, and Roman Medicine: Fifth Century BCE to Third Century CE

1. Homer, *Iliad* IV, 192–219.

2. *Iliad* XI, 825–848.

3. Homer, *Odyssey* XIX, 455.

4. James Longrigg, *Greek Rational Medicine: Philosophy and Medicine from Alcmaeon to the Alexandrians* (London: Routledge, 1993); Werner Wilhelm Jaeger, *Paideia: the Ideals of Greek Culture*, vol. III, trans. Gilbert Highet (New York: Oxford University Press, 1944).

5. W. H. S. Jones, *The Doctor's Oath: An Essay in the History of Medicine* (Cambridge: Cambridge University Press, 1924); Owsei Temkin and C. Lilian Temkin (eds.), *Ancient Medicine: Selected Papers of Ludwig Edelstein* (Baltimore: Johns Hopkins University Press, 1967), pp. 133–144.

6. Karl Deichgraber, *Die Epidemien und das Corpus Hippocraticum* (Berlin, 1933). There are interminable and inconclusive debates over which, if any, of the documents included in the Hippocratic Collection might have been authored by Hippocrates. *Epidemics I* and *Epidemics II* have a better claim to a Hipppocratic provenance than almost any other documents; a good case can also be made for *Aphorisms*.

7. *Epidemics* I, xi, On coctions; Hippocrates, *Ancient Medicine*, xvii, xix, and W. H. S. Jones, "General Introduction," *Hippocrates* (Cambridge: Harvard University Press, 1962), vol. I, pp. li–lii.

8. *Commentary II on Epidemics* I, vii. C. G. Kühn (ed.), *Claudii Galeni Omnia Opera* (Hildesheim: G. Olms, 1964–1965), vol. XVII, pars I, p. 149.

9. Ludwig Edelstein, "The professional ethics of the Greek physician," in Temkin and Temkin, *Ancient Medicine*, p. 324.

10. C. Sandulescu, "Primum non nocere: philological commentaries on a medical aphorism," *Acta Academiae Scientarium Hungaricae* 13 (1965): 359–368.

11. Albert R. Jonsen, "Do no harm: axiom of medical ethics," in Stuart F. Spicker and H. Tristram Englehardt, Jr. (eds.), *Philosophical Medical Ethics: Its Nature and Significance* (Dordrecht: D. Reidel Publishing Company, 1977); Jonsen, "Do no harm," *Annals of Internal Medicine* 88 (1978): 827–832; Diego Gracia Guillén, *Primum Non Nocere. El Principio de No-maleficiencia como Fundamento de la Ética Médica.* (Madrid: Real Acádemia Nacional de Medicina, 1990).

12. *Epidemics* I, xxv.

13. *Prognostic*, section I in *Hippocrates*, vol. II, trans. W. H. S. Jones (Cambridge: Harvard University Press, 1959), p. 9; see "Prognosis" in *Introductory Essays* in *Hippocrates*, vol. II.

14. *Prognostic*, I.

15. "The Art," iii, *Hippocrates*, vol. II, trans. W. H. S. Jones. See "The Art" and "Medical Writing and Laymen," in *Introductory essays*, Hippocrates, vol. II.

16. *The Art*, viii.

17. Vivian Nutton, "Beyond the Hippocratic Oath," in Andrew Wear, Johanna Geyer-Kordesch, and Roger French (eds.), *Doctors and Ethics: The Earlier Historical Setting of Professional Ethics, Clio Medica*, vol. 24 (Amsterdam/Atlanta: Rodopi, 1992), p. 21.

18. Paul Carrick, *Medical Ethics in Antiquity: Philosophical Perspectives on Abortion and Euthanasia* (Dordrecht/Boston: D. Reidel Publishing Company, 1985).

19. Ludwig Edelstein, "The Hippocratic Oath: text, translation and interpretation," in Temkin and Temkin, *Ancient Medicine*, pp. 3–65. The doctrines of Pythagoras and his followers are obscure, although many ancient sources report them in various ways. Among these, Iamblichus, *On the Pythagorean Way of Life*, is the most illuminating (John Dillon and Jackson Hershbell, trans. and eds. [Atlanta: Scholars Press, 1991]). This author describes the concern of the devotees of Pythagoras for spiritual and physical health, attained by exercise and diet. He mentions that the Pythagoreans preferred medical treatment based on diet and that they studied carefully the preparation of foods and its effect on the body; they avoided drugs and surgery (p. 239).

20. Ludwig Edelstein, "The professional ethics of the Greek physician," in Temkin and Temkin, *Ancient Medicine*, pp. 319–348.

21. Nutton, "Beyond the Hippocratic Oath," p. 12; Fridolf Kudlein, "Medical ethics and popular ethics in Greece and Rome," *Clio Medica* 5 (1970): 91–121.

22. Greek philosophical writings do not portray morality as deontological in form, that is, as a morality of rule and precept, but rather as a morality of virtue and aspiration. Still, at the level of popular morality, rule and precept are pervasive, particularly in the belief in a divinely sanctioned, unwritten law (*nomos*), and the binding power of oaths. See Kenneth J. Dover, *Greek Popular Morality in the Time of Plato and Aristotle* (Berkeley: University of California Press, 1974), pp. 246–261.

23. Kudlein, "Medical ethics," pp. 97–107; Temkin and Temkin, *Ancient Medicine*, pp. 11–13.

24. Libanius, *Opera*, vol. VIII, ed. R. Foerster, (Leipzig, 1915), pp. 182–194; Richard M. Ratzan and Gary B. Ferngren, "A Greek progymnasma on the physician-poisoner," *Journal of the History of Medicine and Allied Sciences* 48 (1993): 157–170; see also Darrel W. Amundsen, "The liability of the physician in Greek classical legal theory and practice," *Journal of the History of Medicine and Allied Sciences* 32 (1977): 172–203.

25. Lloyd G. Stevenson, *The Meaning of Poison* (Lawrence: University of Kansas Press, 1959).

26. Aristotle, making a comparison between ethical judgment and medical judgment, notes, "in medicine, it is easy to know what honey, wine and hellebore, cautery and surgery are, but it is difficult to know how, and to whom and when to apply them." Hellebore was a powerful alkaloid, easily harmful, but even wine and honey, when misused, could harm. Aristotle, *Ethics* V, ix, 1137a; also *Magna Moralia* 1199a; see Plato, *Phaedrus*, 268, where Plato also applies the classical rhetorical questions "to whom, when, how much" to the skill of physicians. Maimonides, commenting on the Hippocratic injunction to do no harm, notes that baths, diets, massage with oil, and drinking wine or ice water can be as dangerous as bleeding and purging if done for the wrong conditions or at the wrong times. Suessman Munter (ed.), *The Medical Writings of Moses Maimonides. Treatise on Asthma* (Philadelphia and Montreal: J. B. Lippincott, 1963), pp. 80–81.

27. Markwart Michler, "Medical ethics in Hippocratic bone surgery," *Bulletin of Medical History* 42 (1968): 297–311.

28. Pindar, "Third Pythian Ode," in *Pindar's Victory Songs*, trans. Frank J. Nisetich (Baltimore: Johns Hopkins University Press, 1980).

29. Plato, *Republic* III: 405–407.

30. Ludwig Edelstein, "The professional ethics of the Greek physician," *Bulletin of the History of Medicine* 30 (1956): 392–418; also in Temkin and Temkin, *Ancient Medicine*, pp. 319–348.

31. Aristotle, *Ethics* III, xi, 1119a 16; VI, iv, 1140b11.

32. Kenneth J. Dover, *Greek Popular Morality in the Time of Plato and Aristotle* (Oxford: Blackwell, 1974), pp. 41–45.

33. *Physician*, section I in Jones, trans., *Hippocrates*, vol. II.

34. *Decorum* III.

35. *Decorum* IV.

36. *Precepts* VI.

37. Sir William Osler, *The Old Humanities and the New Science* (Boston/New York: Houghton Mifflin Company, 1920), p. 62.

38. Edelstein, "The professional ethics of the Greek physician"; note *philanthropia* also in Hippocrates, *Physician* I; Galen says that Hippocrates and other ancient physicians healed the sick out of love of mankind, *De Placitis Hippocratis et Platonis*, cited in Temkin and Temkin, *Ancient Medicine*, p. 320.

39. *Decorum* xviii.

40. *Precepts* vi.

41. *Law* V.

42. *Oath*, in Jones, trans., *Hippocrates*, vol. I, p. 229; Heinrich von Staden, "In a pure and holy way. Personal and Professional Conduct in the Hippocratic Oath," *Journal of the History of Medicine and Allied Sciences* 51 (1996): 404–437. Von Staden disputes the theory of Pythagorean origins of Oath and attempts to show by careful linguistic analysis that Oath fits with widespread Greek notions of medicine and religion; he does not shed any light on the exact origins of the document.

43. Jones, trans., *Hippocrates*, vol. II, p. 188.

44. Jones, trans., *Hippocrates*, vol. II, p. 257.

45. Jones, trans., *Hippocrates*, vol. II, pp. 271, 307.

46. Among the numerous references to Hippocratic medicine in Plato, see *Republic* I, 340–342: "No physician, insofar as he is a physician, considers his own good in what he prescribes but the good of his patient"; *Republic* II, 361: "skillful physician, who knows his own powers and keeps within their limits"; *Republic* III, 389: "a lie is useful only as medicine to men and so should be restricted only to physicians (and to statesman)"; *Phaedrus*, 270: "Hippocrates the Asclepiad says the nature of the body can be understood only as a whole"; *Statesman*, pp. 295–299, is a comparison between physician and statesman; *Timeus*, 73–89 is a small treatise on medicine. For medicine in the works of Aristotle, see Werner Jaeger, *Paideia* (New York: Oxford University Press 1962), vol. III, Chapter 1, pp. 3–45. On medicine among the Stoic and Epicurean philosophers, see Martha C. Nussbaum, *The Therapy of Desire: Theory and Practice in Hellenistic Ethics* (Princeton: Princeton University Press, 1994).

47. Andre Bonnard, *Greek Civilization*, vol. II, trans. A. Lytton Sells (New York: The Macmillan Company, 1962), p. 170.

48. Thucydides, *Peloponnesian War*, 2.47.4.

49. *Pseudapigrypha* 5, 3; Owsei Temkin, *Hippocrates in a World of Pagans and Christians* (Baltimore: Johns Hopkins University Press, 1991), p. 58.

50. *Oath* in Jones, trans., *Hippocrates*.

51. *Law* I, in Jones, trans., *Hippocrates*, vol. II, *Precepts* viii.

52. *Precepts* vii.

53. Temkin, *Hippocrates in a World of Pagans*, pp. 80–81; Nutton, "Beyond the Hippocratic Oath," p. 29, n. 8.

54. Plato, *Laws* XI, 933; Aristotle, *Politics* III, 11, 1282a; see Darrel W. Amundsen, "The liability of the physician in classical Greek legal theory and practice," *Journal of the History of Medicine and Allied Sciences* 32 (1977): 172–203.

55. John Scarborough, *Roman Medicine* (Ithaca: Cornell University Press, 1969), p. 41. See also Clifford Allbutt, *Greek Medicine in Rome* (London: Macmillan Company, 1921).

56. Celsus, "Proemium," in *De Medicina*, trans. W. G. Spencer (Cambridge: Harvard University Press, 1960).

57. Vivian Nutton, "Beyond the Hippocratic Oath," in Andrew Wear, Johanna Geyer-Kordesch, and Roger French (eds.), *Doctors and Ethics: The Earlier Historical Setting of Professional Ethics, Clio Medica,* vol. 24 (Amsterdam/Atlanta: Rodopi, 1992).

58. Celsus, *De Medicina*, 3 vols. trans. W. G. Spencer,; Pliny, *Natural History*, 10 vols., trans. W. H. S. Jones (Cambridge: Harvard University Press, 1963).

59. Scribonius Largus, *Compositiones*, in Edmund D. Pellegrino and Alice A. Pellegrino, "Humanism and ethics in Roman medicine: translation and commentary on a text of Scribonius Largus," *Literature and Medicine* 7 (1988): 22–38, p. 26; see also J. S. Hamilton, "Scribonius Largus on the medical profession," *Bulletin of the History of Medicine* 60 (1986): 209–216. The critical edition is Karl Diechgraber, *Professio Medici: Vorwort des Scribonius Largus* (Mainz: Akademie der Wissenschaften, 1950).

60. A similar sentiment is found in a poem about the physician's duty inscribed on a monument set up in the Asklepieion of Athens two centuries after the time Scribonius wrote. "A physician should be like a God, savior equally of slaves, of paupers, of the rich and rulers, and to all a brother giving help." The monument is in honor of a certain Sarapion, described as a Stoic philosopher and physician. J. H. Oliver, "An ancient poem on the duties of a physician," *Bulletin of the History of Medicine* 7 (1935): 315–323.

61. Galen, "The best doctor is a philosopher" in P. N. Singer (trans. and ed.), *Galen: Selected Works* (Oxford: Oxford University Press, 1997), pp. 30–34, p. 33. The standard scholarly edition of Galen is C. G. Kühn (ed.), *Claudii Galeni Opera Omnia* (Hildesheim: Georg Olms, 1965, originally published in 1821–1833); "Optimus medicus" appears in vol. XIV, p. 614. On Galen and his powerful influence on medical knowledge and Western culture in general, see Oswei Temkin, *Galenism: The Rise and Decline of a Medical Philosophy* (London: Cornell University Press, 1973).

62. Nutton, "Beyond the Hippocratic Oath," p. 21.

63. Tacitus, *Annales*, XII, 67; Pliny, *Natural History*, XXIX, 14; *Natural History*, XXIX, 8, 20; Martial, *Epigram* 5.9.

64. *Oxford English Dictionary*, 2d ed. (Oxford: Oxford University Press, 1991).

65. M. Tulli Cicero, *De Officiis*, I, 27.

66. Darrel W. Amundsen, "Murders and miracles: lay attitudes toward medicine in classical antiquity," *Journal of Popular Culture* 11 (1977): 642–655; Fridolf Kudlein, "Medical ethics and popular ethics in Greece and Rome," *Clio Medica* 3 (1970): 91–121.

67. Darrel W. Amundsen, "The liability of physicians in Roman law," in H. Karpus (ed.), *International Symposium on Society, Medicine and Law* (New York: Elsevier Scientific Publishing, 1973), pp. 17–30.

68. Vivian Nutton, "Continuity or rediscovery? The city physician in classical antiquity and medieval Italy," in Andrew W. Russell (ed.), *The Town and State Physician from the Middle Ages to the Enlightenment* (Wolfenbuttel: Herzog August Bibliothek, 1981), pp. 17–21.

69. Vivian Nutton, "Two notes on immunities: *Digest 27*, 1, 6, 10, and 11," *Journal of Roman Studies* 61 (1971): 52–63.

2. Medieval Medicine: Fifth to Fourteenth Centuries CE

1. Owsei Temkin, "History of Hippocratism in late antiquity: the third century and the Latin West," in Owsei Temkin, *The Double Face of Janus and Other Essays in*

the History of Medicine (Baltimore: Johns Hopkins University Press, 1977), pp. 167–177.

2. Owsei Temkin, "Studies on late Alexandrian medicine" and "Byzantine medicine: tradition and empiricism," in Temkin, *The Double Face of Janus*. The monastic medical tradition remains elusive: the libraries of ninth- and tenth-century European monasteries contained many, often garbled classical texts, although some, like the Hippocratic *Prognostic*, were preserved rather well. See Loren C. McKinney, "Medical ethics and etiquette in the Early Middle Ages: the persistence of Hippocratic ideals," *Bulletin of the History of Medicine* 6 (1952): 1–31; Pearl Kibre, *Hippocrates Latinus: Repertorium of Hippocratic Writings in the Latin Middle Ages* (New York: Fordham University Press, 1985); Frederick Paxton, "*Signa Mortifera*: death and prognostication in early medieval monastic medicine," *Bulletin of the History of Medicine* 67 (1993): 631–650.

3. St. Basil, "The Long Rule," in St. Basil, *Ascetical Works*, trans. M. M. Wagner (Washington, D.C.: The Catholic University of America Press, 1950), Rule 55. See Darrel W. Amundsen, "Medicine and faith in early Christianity," *Bulletin of the History of Medicine*, 56 (1982): 326–350.

4. Temkin, *Hippocrates in a World of Pagans and Christians*, p. 144.

5. Luke 10: 29–37. It has been noted that 727 of the 3779 verses of the four New Testament Gospels pertain to the healing of physical or mental illness or the resurrection of the dead. S. G. Post, "Baby K: medical futility and the freedom of religion," *Journal of Law, Medicine, and Ethics* 23 (1995): 20–26.

6. "Homily 10 on Hebrews 6, 7–8" in Philip Schaff (ed.), *The Nicene and Post-Nicene Fathers of the Christian Church*, series 1 (New York: Charles Scribner's Sons, 1905–1908), XIV, p. 417.

7. Rodney Stark, *The Rise of Christianity* (San Francisco: HarperCollins, 1997), pp. 76–94. Citations from Cyprian ("On Mortality," 15–20), Dionysius ("Festival Letters" in Eusebius, *Ecclesiastical History*, 7.22), and Julian ("Letter 49") are taken from this book, pp. 81, 83, 84.

8. Gregory Nazienzus, "Panegyric on Saint Basil," Oration XLIII, 63, in Schaff, *Nicene and Post-Nicene Fathers*, series 2, Vol. VII, p. 126.

9. Temkin, *Hippocrates in a World of Pagans and Christians*, ch. 12.

10. Cassiodorus Senator, *An Introduction to Divine and Human Readings*, trans. Leslie Jones (New York: Columbia University Press, 1946).

11. Hildegard also wrote a general treatise on medical diagnosis and treatment, *Causae et Curae*. On the life of this extraordinary woman, see Sabina Flanagan, *Hildegard of Bingen. A Visionary Life* (New York: Routledge, 1989). Relatively little has been written on the medical and pharmaceutical works of Hildegard; a short treatment can be found in Kate Hurd-Mead, *A History of Women in Medicine* (Boston: Milford House, 1938), pp. 183–194, and a more extensive exposition appears in Anton Brück (ed.), *Hildegard von Bingen* (Mainz: Gesellschaft für MittleRheinischer Kirchengeschichte, 1979).

12. Fulbert's *Hymnus de Sancto Pantaleone* is cited in Loren C. MacKinney, *Early Medieval Medicine* (Baltimore: Johns Hopkins University Press, 1937), p. 134. MacKinney tells the story of Bishop Derold in "Tenth century medicine as seen in the Historia of Richter of Rheims," *Bulletin of the Institute of the History of Medicine* 2 (1034): 347–375.

13. The phrase "Our lords, the sick" is the common designation of the patients served by the Hospitallers and appears in the first known rule of the Order, dating probably from 1153. The complaint of the hospital administrator is cited in Jonathan Riley-Smith, *The Knights of Saint John in Jerusalem and Cyprus* (New York: Macmillan Company, 1976), p. 331. See also H. J. A. Shire, *The Knights of Malta* (New Haven: Yale University Press,

1994); Edgar Erskine Hume, *The Medical Work of the Knights Hospitallers of St. John and the Hospitals of the West* (Baltimore: Johns Hopkins University Press, 1940); Timothy Miller, "The Knights of St. John and the hospitals of the West," *Speculum* 53 (1978): 709–733. Although the Knights and the Saracens were fierce enemies in battle, there was mutual respect, particularly regarding hospital work. One historian notes, "The tolerance of the Muslims regarding the Hospital was doubtless inspired by the fact that, from their origin, the Hospitallers adopted as a principle the welcome of all the sick needing care, whether Muhammadans, Christians or Jews." Prosper Jardin, *Les Chevalier de Malte* (Paris: Librarie Academique Perrin, 1974), p. 41. Legend has it that Sulieman the Magnificent received care at a hospital of the Knights.

14. Antoine Leal, *Le chevalier de Saint Jean de Jerusalem ou L'idee parfaite du religieux hospitalier militant*, MS, Marseille, 1616, in the Archives of the Knights of Malta, Rome. On the militant religious orders, see Desmond Seward, *The Monks of War* (London: Penguin Books, 1972).

15. Cited in Temkin, *Hippocrates in a World of Pagans and Christians*, p. 182.

16. Jerome, "Letter III to Nepotianus," in F. A. Wright (ed.), *Select Letters of St. Jerome* (London: W. Heinemann, Ltd., 1933), letter 52, p. 225.

17. Edinburgh A.5.42, twelfth century, last folio, quoted in Loren C. MacKinney, "Medical ethics and etiquette in the early middle ages: the persistence of Hippocratic ideals," *Bulletin of the History of Medicine* 26 (1952): 1–31, quote on p. 15.

18. Chartres MS, 62, tenth-century folios 1–2, quoted in MacKinney, "Medical ethics," p. 12; St. Gall, 751, ninth-tenth centuries, quoted in MacKinney, "Medical ethics," p. 19; Urbanus 64, folio 116. The earliest manuscript of the Hippocratic Oath is Vindobonensis med IV, tenth century. The Christian version can be read in Jones, *The Doctor's Oath*, pp. 22–26. The major change in the Christian version, apart from a new deity, is a stronger statement about abortion, which now reads "I will not give women treatment to cause abortion, either from above or below" (i.e., by oral drugs or by surgical manipulation).

19. Robert M. Veatch and Carol G. Mason, "Hippocratic vs. Judeo-Christian medical ethics: principles in conflict," *Journal of Religious Ethics* 15 (1986): 86–105; Carlos Calvão-Sabrihno, "Hippocratic ideals, medical ethics and the practice of medicine in the early middle ages: legacy of the Hippocratic Oath," *Journal of the History of Medicine and Allied Sciences* 50 (1996), 438–456.

20. Lateran Council IV, chapters 21 and 22, in Henry Denzinger and Adolf Schonmetzer (eds.), *Enchiridion Symbolorum Definitionum et Declarationum De Rebus Fidei et Morum* (Rome: Herder Verlag, 1965), 33rd ed., pp. 812–815; Darrel W. Amundsen, "The Medieval Catholic tradition" in Ronald L. Numbers and Amundsen (eds.), *Caring and Curing: Health and Medicine in the Western Religious Tradition* (New York: Macmillan Company, 1986), pp. 84–91.

21. Darrel W. Amundsen, "Casuistry and professional obligations: the regulation of physicians by the court of conscience in the late Middle Ages," *Transactions and Studies of the College of Physicians of Philadelphia* 3 (1981): 22–39, 93–112.

22. John T. Noonan, Jr., "An almost absolute value in history," in Noonan (ed.), *The Morality of Abortion: Legal and Historical Perspectives* (Cambridge: Harvard University Press, 1970); John T. Noonan, Jr., *Contraception* (Cambridge: Harvard University Press, 1970).

23. Edinburgh MS A.5.42, in MacKinney, "Medical ethics," p. 15.

24. Constantinus Africanus, Prologue, *Liber Pantegni*, MacKinney, "Medical ethics," p. 31.

25. Thomas Aquinas, *Summa Theologiae* II-II, Q. 71, a.7.

26 "Henri de Mondeville on the morals and etiquette of surgeons" in Stanley Joel Reiser, Arthur J. Dyck, and William J. Curran (eds.), *Ethics in Medicine: Historical Perspectives and Contemporary Concerns* (Cambridge: MIT Press, 1977), p. 15, from D'Arcy Power (ed.) *Treatises de Fistula in Ano* (London: Kegan Paul, Trench, Trubner and Co., Ltd., 1910) pp. xx–xxii.

27. Donald Campbell, *Arabian Medicine and Its Influence on the Middle Ages*, 2 vols. (London: Kegan Paul, Trench, Trubner, 1926).

28. Cyril Lloyd Elgood, *A Medical History of Persia and the Eastern Caliphate from the Earliest Times until the Year A.D. 1932* (Cambridge: Cambridge University Press, 1951), p. 52. On Jundi-Shapur, see Allen O. Whipple, *The Role of Nestorians and Muslims in the History of Medicine* (Princeton: Princeton University Press, 1966), and Allen O. Whipple, "The role of the Nestorians as the connecting link between Greek and Arab medicine," *Annals of Medical History* 8 (1936): 313–323. The sole remnants of this stellar institution are several tumuli that have not been excavated, near the village of Shahadbad in the southwestern corner of Iran. Roy Porter notes that "there is no evidence that any medical academy existed there (at Jundi-shapur)" (*The Greatest Benefit to Mankind*, p. 94). This assertion is remarkable, since major historians of Arabic medicine attest to intensive medical scholarship and the existence of the bimaristan. Some of the language in the above text comes from my own editing of Abdulaziz Sachedina, "Medical ethics, history of: Near and Middle East, Iran," in Warren Reich, *Encyclopedia of Bioethics* (New York: Simon & Schuster, 1995), vol. III, pp. 1445–1449.

29. Martin Levey, *Medical Ethics of Medieval Islam: With Special Reference to Al-Ruhawi's Practical Ethics of the Physician* (Philadelphia: American Philosophical Society, 1967), pp. 93, 94, 71. Strangely enough, Al-Ruhawi may have been a Christian (Levey, p. 8). He was apparently from Edessa, which was a major center of Nestorian scholarship. If he was a Christian, no sign of that faith appears in the text, which opens with the usual Islamic doxology, "In the name of Allah, the beneficent and compassionate, in whom I have trust and for whose help I ask" (Levey, p. 18), and all theological references are in the Islamic idiom. He may have been raised as a Nestorian Christian. Since that sectarian belief maintained only a tenuous association between the Divine Logos and the man Jesus, it may have been relatively easy for Nestorians to slip from trinitarian Christianity into monotheistic Islam. Whatever his faith, he sounds like a Muslim from the beginning to the end of his treatise.

30. O. Cameron Gruner (trans.), *A Treatise on the Canon of Medicine of Avicenna, Incorporating a Translation of the First Book* (New York: Augustus Kelly, 1970), sections 27–28.

31. Hakim Mohammed Said, *Al-Tibb Al-Islam. A Brief Survey of the Development of Tibb (Medicine) during the Days of the Holy Prophet Mohammad and in the Islamic Age* (Karachi: Hamdard National Foundation, 1979), pp. 88–99. Also Abdulaziz Sachedina, Nil Sari, and Hassan Hathout, "Medical ethics, history of, Near and Middle East," in Reich (ed.), *Encyclopedia of Bioethics*, vol. III, pp. 1445–1457; Fazlur Rahman, *Health and Medicine in the Islamic Tradition* (New York: Crossroad, 1989); Donald Campbell, *Arabian Medicine and Its Influences on the Middle Ages* (London: Kegan Paul, Trench, Trubner and Co., Ltd., 1926).

32. Ecclus. 38:1; Darrel W. Amundsen, "Medicine and faith in early Christianity," *Bulletin of the History of Medicine* 56 (1982): 326–350; Sir Immanuel Jakobovits, *Jewish Medical Ethics: A Comparative and Historical Study of the Jewish Religious Attitude to Medicine and Its Practice* (New York: Bloch Publishing Company, 1959), ch. 1; Temkin, *Hippocrates in a World of Pagans and Christians*, pp. 88–93.

33. Isaac Israeli, *Propedeutic for Physicians*, trans. Martin Levey, in *Transactions of the American Philosophical Society* NS 57; 3 (1967): 95–97. See David Margalith, "The ideal doctor as depicted in ancient Hebrew writings," *Journal of History of Medicine and Allied Health Sciences* (1953) 12: 37–41. The closing words of this citation become common coin in Renaissance ethics treatises.

34. Maimonides, Hillel Shabbath, ii, 3; Mishneh Torah, Hilchot Rotze'ach 114; Mishneh Torah, Hilchot Rotze'ach, 1:9; Mishneh Torah, Hilchot Avel, 4:5; Munter (ed.), *The Medical Writings of Moses Maimonides. Treatise on Asthma*, p. 89; Ariel Bar-Sela and Hebble Hoff, "Interpretation of the First Aphorism of Hippocrates," *Bulletin of the History of Medicine* 37 (1963): 347–354, p. 354.

35. David Reisman, *The Story of Medicine in the Middle Ages* (New York: Paul Hoeber, 1936), p. 67; David M. Feldman, *Health and Medicine in the Jewish Tradition* (New York: Crossroad, 1986); Harry Friedenwald *The Jews and Medicine* (Baltimore: Johns Hopkins University Press, 1944). Texts from Azwazi, Asaph, and the Prayer of Maimonides and others are printed in the Appendix, *Encyclopedia of Bioethics* (New York: Simon & Schuster, 1995), vol. V, pp. 2633–2639. It should be noted, however, that the beautiful "Physician's Prayer" attributed to Maimonides was actually written by a German Jewish physician, Marcus Herz, about 1793.

36. Reisman, *The Story of Medicine in the Middle Ages*, ch. VI; Nancy Siraisi, *Medieval and Early Renaissance Medicine* (Chicago: University of Chicago Press, 1990), pp. 29–31, 50–51. In Spain during the twelfth and thirteen centuries, there was a particularly vital communication between Christian and Jewish physicians who used Arabic as a common learned language. See Luis García-Ballester, "A marginal learned world: Jewish, Muslim and Christian medical practitioners, and the use of Arabic medical sources in late medieval Spain," in Luis García-Ballester, Roger French, Jon Arrizabalaga, and Andrew Cunningham, *Practical Medicine from Salerno to the Black Death* (Cambridge: Cambridge University Press, 1994), pp. 353–395.

37. The origins of medical activities at Salerno are unclear. Constantinus Africanus' work seems to have been done several decades before the appearance of any sort of medical teaching in the city. Among the mysteries surrounding Salerno is the alleged presence of women as teachers and students, particularly a famous but elusive Trotula, who authored a treatise on the diseases of women. See Paul Kristeller, "The school of Salerno. Its development and contribution to the history of learning," *Bulletin of the History of Medicine* 17 (1945): 138–194, and Luis García-Ballester "Introduction," in García-Ballester et al., *Practical Medicine*, pp. 13–29.

38. Guglielmo da Saliceto, *Cirurgia* II.5, cited in Jole Agrimi and Chiara Crisciani, "The Science and practice of medicine in the thirteenth century according to Guglielmo da Saliceto, Italian surgeon," in García-Ballester et al., *Practical Medicine*, pp. 60–87, p. 77.

39. Frederick II, "Medieval law for the regulation of the practice of medicine," in Stanley Joel Reiser, Arthur J. Dyck, and William J. Curran (eds.), *Ethics in Medicine: Historical Perspectives and Contemporary Concerns* (Cambridge: MIT Press, 1977), pp. 10–12.

40. Vern L. Bullough, *The Development of Medicine as a Profession* (New York: Hafner, 1966); on guilds, see Richard MacKenney, *Tradesmen and Trades: The World of the Guild in Venice and Europe, c. 1250–c. 1650* (London: Routledge, 1990). Pope John XXII, whose prepapal name was Peter of Spain, had been a renowned practitioner of medicine, particularly in ophthalmology. He wrote *The Treasury of the Poor*, a widely appreciated medical treatise for those who could not afford doctors' fees.

41. Darrel Amundsen, "Medical ethics, history of: Europe," in Reich (ed.), *The Encyclopedia of Bioethics*, vol. 3, p. 1527.

42. On the conflict between altruism and self-interest, see Albert R. Jonsen, *The New Medicine and the Old Ethics* (Cambridge: Harvard University Press, 1990). The relationship between professions and self-interest is expounded in many books, among them Jeffrey L. Berlant, *Profession and Monopoly: A Study of Medicine in the United States and Great Britain* (Berkeley and Los Angeles: University of California Press, 1975).

43. Hippocrates, *Aphorisms. Hippocrates with an English Translation*, trans. W. H. S. Jones, (Cambridge: Harvard University Press, 1959), vol. IV, p. 99; Dickenson W. Richards, "The First Aphorism of Hippocrates," *Perspectives in Biology and Medicine* (1961), 5: 61–64. Innumerable commentaries have been written on these few words. Galen wrote a magisterial commentary, as did Maimonides (Galen, *Hippocrates Aphorismi et Galeni in eos Commentarii*, in C. G. Kühn [ed.], *Claudii Galeni Opera Omnia*, XVII, 345–355 [Hildesheim: Georg Olms, 1965], p. 346); Ariel Bar-Sela and Hebbel Hoff, "Maimonides' interpretation of the First Aphorism of Hippocrates," *Bulletin of the History of Medicine* (1963) 37: 347–357; Franz Rosenthal, "'Life is short, the Art is long': Arabic commentaries on the First Hippocratic Aphorism," *Bulletin of the History of Medicine* 40 (1966): 226–245. Hippocrates' words about medicine evoke reflections on life itself, and the text has even been used by theologians and mystics: see Diego Gracia, "Hipócrates a lo Divino," in *Historia y Medicina en España* (Valladolid: Junta de Castilla y Leon, 1994), pp. 57–77.

44. *Explicatio super Canonem Vita Brevis* in *Arnaldi Villanova Opera Omnia* (Basil: Ex Officina Pernea, 1585), col. 1710. Vilanova's second treatise, written as an outline of comments on the aphorism, is *Tabula super Vita Brevis*, and the treatise on the ethics of urinoscopy is *De Cautelis Medicorum* (Opera Omnia, col. 1453), anthologized in Reiser et al., pp. 12–15, quote on page 13. A modern critical edition of the works of Vilanova is being prepared, but volume IV, which contains these treatises, is not yet in print (Michael McVaugh [ed.], *Arnaldi de Vilanova Opera Medica Omnia* [Barcelona: Universitat de Barcelona]). On de Vilanova's medical ethics, see García-Ballester, "Medical ethics in transition in the Latin medicine of the thirteenth and fourteenth centuries: new perspectives on the physician-patient relationship and the doctor's fee" in Wear et al., *Doctors and Ethics*, pp. 38–71.

45. Guy de Chauliac, *La Grande Chirurgie*, ed. and trans. into French by E. Nicaise (Paris: Felix Alcan, 1890), p. 19, cited in Bullough, *The Development of Medicine as a Profession*, p. 94.

3. Medical Ethics of India and China

1. Bhagvat Sinh Jee, *A Short History of Aryan Medical Science* (Gondal: Shree Bhagvat Sinh Jee Electric Press, 1927), p. 27. The Ashvini appear in Rig Veda I, 117, 13. The story of the decapitation is told rather differently in other texts; in *Caraka Samhita* the Ashvini twins teach Indra, not vice versa. In *Taittiriya Samhita* 6.9.1 it is specifically stated that physicians, because of their impurity, are excluded from the sacrifices and that Brahmans must not practice medicine. See Kenneth G. Zysk, *Asceticism and Healing in Ancient India* (New York and Oxford: Oxford University Press, 1991), pp. 22–23.

2. *Manu-Smrti* in Louis Renou, *Hinduism* (New York: George Braziller, 1962), pp. 116–130.

3. Prakash Desai, *Health and Medicine in the Hindu Tradition: Continuity and Cohesion* (New York: Crossroads, 1989). For a brief overview of the Hindu tradition of medical ethics, see Prakash Desai, "Medical ethics, history of: South and East Asia, India," in

Reich (ed.), *Encyclopedia of Bioethics*, 1995, vol. III, pp. 1471–1477, and A. L. Basham and Mitchell Weiss, "Hinduism," in Reich, *Encyclopedia of Bioethics*, vol. II, pp. 1132–1139. Standard expositions of ancient Indian medicine are Jean Filliozat, *La doctrine classique de la médicine indienne, ses origines et ses parallèles grecs* (Paris: Imprimerie Nationale, 1949), and Julius Jolly, *Indian Medicine* (New Delhi: Munshiram Manoharlal, 1977).

4. Kenneth Zysk, in *Asceticism and Healing in Ancient India*, proposes the controversial but convincing thesis that ayurvedic medicine was the creation of heterodox wandering ascetics who lived and worked outside orthodox Brahman society. These Hindu ascetics, who could mingle freely with all castes, were compatible with the earliest Buddhist monks, and together they formulated what later became the Hindu *ayurveda*.

5. *Agnivesa's Caraka Samhita*, Ram Sharma and B. Dash, trans. and eds. (Varanasi: Chowkhamba Sanskrit Series Office, 1976), Vol. I, ch. vii, pp. 171–173; ch. xxix, pp. 587–591; see also ch. xxx, pp. 617–619, where the ignorant physician is called "the noose of death." The "therapeutic exception" is not in the text of the *Caraka Samhita*, but in the classical commentary of Cakrapani (eleventh century), who offers the case of a patient who should eat crow meat, which he despises; the physician may tell him it is partridge. *Caraka Samhita*, ch. viii, p. 175.

6. *Charaka Samhita* (Jamnagar, India: Shree Galbkuverba Ayurvedic Society, 1947), Vol. 5, p. 326. This oath is printed in Reich (ed.), *The Encyclopedia of Bioethics*, vol. 5, p. 2632. See A. Menon and H. F. Haberman, "A medical students' oath of ancient India," *Medical History* 14 (1970): 295. The opening words of the oath enjoin celibacy and poverty, which suggests the origin of *ayurveda* among Hindu ascetics and possibly the requirements for novice physicians. Menon and Haberman speculate about the influence of this oath on the Hippocratic Oath through the Pythangorean connection to Indian thought.

7. Renou, *Hinduism*, p. 56.

8. *Mahavagga*, 8.26.3.

9. On the relationship of ayurvedic medicine and Buddhist thought and practice, see Zysk, *Asceticism and Healing in Ancient India*.

10. Among the many histories of Chinese medicine, the most accessible and readable is Paul Unschuld's *Medicine in China: A History of Ideas* (Berkeley: University of California Press, 1985). Joseph Needham's *Science and Civilization in China* (Cambridge: Cambridge University Press, 1954–) is a fascinating and astonishingly learned exploration of Chinese history and culture. The section dealing with medicine is not yet in print but is promised in 2000 (Joseph Needham, with Lu Gwei-djen, *Science and Civilization in China*, vol. 6, part 6, with an Introduction by Nathan Siven). Much of the material that will appear in this volume can be found in three succinct, insightful, and informative essays: Joseph Needam, "Medicine and Chinese culture," "Hygiene and preventive medicine in ancient China," and "China and the origin of qualifying examinations in medicine," in Needham, *Clerks and Craftsmen in China and the West* (Cambridge: Cambridge University Press, 1970), pp. 263–287, 340–378, 379–395. On the history of acupuncture and moxibustion, see Lu Gwei-djen and Joseph Needham, *Celestial Lancets* (Cambridge: Cambridge University Press, 1980). On the vast pharmacology and materia medica of traditional Chinese medicine, see Paul Unschuld, *Medicine in China. A History of Pharmaceutics* (Berkeley and Los Angeles: University of California Press, 1986).

11. Simon Leyes, (trans.) *The Analects of Confucius* (New York: W.W. Norton, 1997), 1.2, p. 3. The words are quoted as those of Master You Ruo, one of Confucius' two principal disciples, but they certainly reflect, with remarkable succinctness, the Master's central thought. It might be noted that the virtue of filial piety (*xiao*) and concomitant obedi-

ence to authority was emphasized by the imperial rulers out of proportion to its place in the total thought of the Master. See Leyes, pp. 134–135.

12. Ilza Vieth (transl. and ed.), *Huang Ti Nei Ching Su Wen. The Yellow Emperor's Classic of Internal Medicine* (Berkeley and Los Angeles: University of California Press, 1966). Needham calls this work "a counterpart of the Hippocratic Corpus, not quite so old but not very much younger; and no less rational than the best medical thought of the Greek and Hellenistic worlds" (*Celestial Lancets*, p. xviii). The common English title of this work, *Internal Medicine*, is misleading: it has nothing to do with the modern medical specialty of the same name. Needham suggests that the word *nei*, which means "inner," as distinguished from "outer," refers in this context to "everything this-wordly, rational, practical, concrete, repeatable, verfiable, in other words, scientific. Similarly, *wai* or 'outside' means everything other-wordly, everything to do with gods and spirits, sages and immortals, everything exceptional, miraculous, strange, uncanny, unearthly, extra-mundane and extra-corporeal." Needham prefers the translation *Corporeal Medicine*. I have taken a middle path, using *Inner*. Joseph Needham, "Medicine and Chinese culture," in *Clerks and Craftsmen in China and the West*, pp. 263–297, p. 272. The Pinyin system for romanization of Chinese words is used in the text of this book; in the endnotes, the system found in the original citation is retained.

13. Vieth, Introduction, on p. 10; *Nei Ching*, Book I, I, p. 97. It is intriguing that the Indian *Caraka Samhita* opens with a convention of sages inquiring into the impediments to longevity. *Caraka Samhita*, ch. 1, pp. 16–26.

14. Vieth, *Nei Ching*, Bk. I, ch. 2, p. 105. This text is quoted in Unschuld, *Medicine in China: A History of Ideas*, p. 63. Unschuld's footnote recalls an analogous passage from Eristratos, quoted by Edelstein (in Temkin and Temkin, *Ancient Medicine*, p. 307), and I am reminded of Plato's discussion of *Asklepios politicos*.

15. Unshuld, *Medical Ethics in Imperial China* (Berkeley and Los Angeles: University of California Press, 1979), p. 37, citing Kao Pao-Cheng, Preface to *Chia-i ching*, c. +1092. Unshuld's book contains translations of all the major extant texts on Chinese medical ethics from the sixth to the nineteenth century CE. For a brief overview of the long tradition of Chinese medical ethics, see Unschuld, "Medical Ethics, history of, South and East Asia, Pre-Republican China," in Reich (ed.), *Encyclopedia of Bioethics* vol. III, pp. 1477–1483.

16. Vieth, p. 87, citing Wang Pin, "Introduction" to the *Enlarged Edition of Nei Ching*. Wang Pin is more than a commentator; in +762, he claimed to have rediscovered and restored the original text, much of which had been lost and the remainder corrupted.

17. Archie J. Bahm (trans.), *Tao Teh King* by Lao Tzu (Albuquerque: World Books, 1958), I, XXI, LXVII, pp. 11, 26, 60.

18. Unshuld, *Medical Ethics*, p. 143, citing a first-century CE Buddhist medical text.

19. A fine exposition of Confucian, Neo-Confucian, Buddhist, and Taoist thought, especially in relation to science and medicine, can be found in Needham, *Science and Civilization in China*, vol. 2.

20. Unschuld, *Medical Ethics*, p. 57, citing Yu Pien, *Hsu i-shou* (+1522).

21. Unschuld, *Medical Ethics*, p. 28.

22. Kenneth K. S. Ch'en, *Buddhism in China. A Historical Survey* (Princeton: Princeton University Press, 1964). Vast numbers of monks and nuns were secularized during this brief suppression, but a subsequent emperor, who was himself a Buddhist devotee, ordered an equally vast ordination to restore the ranks of the Buddhist clergy.

23. Needham, "Qualifying examinations," in *Clerks and Craftsmen*, pp. 379–395.

24. Unshuld, *Medical Ethics*, pp. 30–33, citing Sun Ssu-miao (+581–682), *Ch'ien-chin fang*. Sun Ssu-miao also wrote a later work in which he included a chapter on moral

duties apparently excerpted from a much earlier medical text. However, it appears to be an exortation to all persons, rather than just to practitioners of medicine, and reflects a mix of Buddhist and Taoist beliefs.

25. Unshuld, *Medical Ethics*, p. 35.

26. Unshuld, *Medical Ethics*, p. 37, citing K'ou Tsung-shih (c. +1119), *Pen-ts'ao yen-i*.

27. Unshuld, *Medical Ethics*, pp. 44–53, citing Chiang Ch'ou (c. +1207), *I-shou*.

28. Unshuld, *Medical Ethics*, p. 74, citing Kung T'ing-hsien (c. +1615), *Wan-ping hui-ch'un*.

29. Unshuld, *Medical Ethics*, pp. 101–102. "Warnings to physicians" is part of the author's larger medical treatise, *Ku-chin i-che* (+1808).

30. Ralph C. Crozier, *Traditional Medicine in Modern China: Science, Nationalism and Cultural Change* (Cambridge: Harvard University Press, 1968), p. 107. For a brief overview of the evolution of medical ethics in postimperial China, see Ren-zong Qiu and Albert Jonsen, "Medical ethics, history of, South and East Asia: contemporary China," in Reich (ed.), *Encyclopedia of Bioethics*, vol. III, pp. 1483–1490. I have, with Dr. Qiu's gracious permission, borrowed some words from this article.

31. Song Guo-bin, *Ethics of Medical Practice* (Shanghai: Guoguang Bookstore, 1933).

32. Hippocrates, Precepts X; Lu Chih, *Ch'ien-chin fang*, cited in Unschuld, *Medical Ethics*, p. 35.

33. Veith, *Nei Ching*, I, 4, p. 113.

4. Renaissance and Enlightenment: Fourteenth to Eighteenth Centuries

1. See Winfried Schleiner, *Medical Ethics in the Renaissance* (Washingon, D.C.: Georgetown University Press, 1995); Andrew Wear, Roger French, and I. M. Lonie, *The Medical Renaissance of the Sixteenth Century* (Cambridge: Cambridge University Press, 1985). The quote from Yperman is from his *De cyryrgie*, Book I, ch. iv, cited in Bullough, *The Development of Medicine as a Profession*, p. 95.

2. Luis García-Ballester, "Medical ethics in transition. Latin medicine in the thirteenth and fourteenth centuries: new problems in the physician–patient relationship and with the doctor's fee," in Wear et al., *Doctors and Ethics*, p. 45.

3. Henri de Mondeville, cited in Reiser et al., *Ethics in Medicine*, p. 15.

4. Thomas Aquinas, *In Octo Libros Politicorum Aristotelis Expositio*, I, viii. ed. R. Spiazzi (Turin and Rome: Marietti 1966).

5. Richard Palmer, "Physicians and the state in post-medieval Italy," in Andrew Russell (ed.), *The Town and State Physician in Europe from the Middle Ages to the Enlightenment* (Wolfenbüttel: Herzog August Bibliothek, 1981), pp. 47–62; Carlos M. Cipolla, *Cristofano and the Plague: A Study in the History of Public Health in the Age of Galileo* (Berkeley and Los Angeles: University of California Press, 1973) and *Public Health and the Medical Profession in the Renaissance* (Cambridge: Cambridge University Press, 1976). On the duty to care for plague victims, see Darrel W. Amundsen, "Medical deontology and pestilential disease in the late Middle Ages," *Journal of the History of Medicine and Allied Sciences* 32 (1977): 403–421; also George Deaux, *The Black Death* (London; Hamilton, 1969), and A. M. Campbell, *The Black Death and Men of Learning* (New York: Columbia University Press, 1931).

6. Ole Peter Grell, "Conflicting duties: plague and the obligations of early modern physicians toward patients and the commonwealth in England and the Netherlands," in Wear et al., *Doctors and Ethics*, pp. 131–152; Martin Luther, *Ob man vor dem Sterben*

fliehen möge (1527); Theodore Beza, *A shorte learned and pithie Treatize of the Plague, wherin are handled these two questions: The one, whether the Plague bee infectious or no: The other, whether and howe farre it may of Christians bee shunned by going outside,* trans. John Stockwood (London: 1580); Marcello Zalba, *Theologiae Moralis Compendium* (Madrid: Biblioteca Autore Cristianos, 1963), II, no. 324; Talmud, Kamma 60B, cited in Immanuel Jakobovits, *Jewish Medical Ethics* (New York: Bloch Publishing, 1959), p. 11.

7. Guy de Chauliac, *La Grande Chirurgie* (Paris: Nicaise, 1890), pp. 171–172.

8. Quoted in C. E. A. Winslow, *The Conquest of Epidemic Disease: A Chapter in the History of Ideas* (Madison: University of Wisconsin Press, 1980), p.118 (first ed. published in 1943 by Princeton Unversity Press).

9. Samuel Pepys, *The Illustrated Pepys: Extracts from the Diary,* ed. Robert Latham (London: Bell and Hyman Ltd., 1978), p. 98. See J. Leasor, *The Plague and the Fire* (New York: Avon Books, 1961).

10. William Boghurst, *Loimographia* (1666) in *Transactions of the Epidemiological Society of London* 13 (1894): 59–60.

11. Daniel Sennert, *De lue venerea,* in Sennert, *Opera Omnia* (Lyon, 1666), vols. 4–5, p. 1014, cited in Schleiner, *Medical Ethics in the Renaissance,* p. 177. On the origins of syphilis, see Claude Quétel, *History of Syphilis,* trans. Judith Braddock and Brian Pike (London: Polity Press, 1990).

12. Cotton Mather, *The Angel of Bethesda,* trans. Gordon W. Jones (Barre, Mass: American Antiquarian Society, 1972), p. 120. Medical views about sexuality were often difficult to reconcile with the views of moralists; see Danielle Jacquart and Claude Thomasset, *Sexuality and Medicine in the Middle Ages,* trans. Matthew Adamson (Princeton: Princeton University Press, 1988).

13. "Agents [in matters of right conduct] are compelled at every step to think out for themselves what the circumstances demand, just as happens in the art of medicine and navigation" (*Nicomachean Ethics,* II, ii, 1104a11; V, ix, 1137a17). The navigation analogy becomes a favorite with early medical writers. For example, Arnau de Vilanova writes, "The physician's duty is like that of the sea-captain . . . based not on necessary rules but on contingencies: the captain trims his sails as the wind shifts, so the doctor should change his treatments as dictated by the condition of the patient." *Super canonem Vita Brevis,* p. 1712.

14. Cicero, *De Officiis,* trans. Walter Miller (Cambridge: Harvard University Press, 1975), III, xxiii, pp. 363–367. Arguments similar to Cicero's (that a lottery should decide) are repeated in Edmond Cahn's *The Moral Decision* (Bloomington, Ind.: Indiana University Press 1955), which becomes a source for many ethicists' analyses of allocation of lifesaving medical technologies; see Jonsen, *The Birth of Bioethics* (New York: Oxford University Press), ch. 7.

15. The distinction between *ordinary* and *extraordinary* was first formulated by the Spanish theologians Dominico Soto and Dominico Banez; see James J. McCartney, "The development of the doctrine of ordinary and extraordinary means of preserving life in Catholic moral theology," *Linacre Quarterly* 47 (1980): 215. One of the earliest and most detailed works of medical-moral theology is Paolo Zacchias, *Quaestiones Medico-Legales* (Rome, 1621–1650). On the history of Catholic moral theology on medicine, see Darrel Amundsen, "Casuistry and professional obligations: the regulation of physicians by the court of conscience in the late Middle Ages," *Transactions and Studies of the College of Physicians of Philadelphia* 1 (1981): 22–39; 2 (1982): 93–112; David F. Kelly, *The Emergence of Roman Catholic Medical Ethics in North America: An Historical-Methodological-*

Bibliographical Study (New York and Toronto: Edwin Mellen Press, 1979). On casuistry in general, see Albert R. Jonsen and Stephen Toulmin, *The Abuse of Casuistry: A History of Moral Reasoning* (Berkeley and Los Angeles: University of California Press, 1986). Moral questions concerning reproduction were prominent in this literature. See, for example, John Connery, *Abortion: The Development of the Roman Catholic Perspective* (Chicago: Loyola University Press, 1977), and John T. Noonan, Jr., *Contraception. A History of Its Treatment by the Catholic Theologians and Canonists* (Cambridge: Harvard University Press, 1965). A fuller treatment of the Renaissance Catholic medical moralists can be found in Schleiner, *Medical Ethics in the Renaissance*.

16. Thomas Aquinas, *Summa theologiae* II-II, q. 65, a. 1; see Joseph Mangan, "An historical analysis of the principle of double effect," *Theological Studies* 10 (1949): 40–61.

17. Giovanni Codronchus, *De Christiana ac Tuta Medendi Ratione* (Frankfurt, 1597), vol. I, p. 43; Ahasverius Fritsch, *Medicus Peccans sive Tractatus de Peccatis Medicorum* (Nuremberg, 1684).

18. L. R. Lind, *Studies in Pre-Vesalian Anatomy: Biography, Translations, Documents* (Philadelphia: American Philosophical Society, 1975), p. 151.

19. Andrew French, "The medical ethics of Gabriele de Zerbi," in Andrew Wear, Roger K. French, and I. M. Lonie (eds.), *The Medical Renaissance of the Sixteenth Century* (Cambridge: Cambridge University Press, 1984), p. 84.

20. French, "The medical ethics of Gabriele de Zerbi," p. 94.

21. Sir George N. Clark, *A History of the Royal College of Physicians of London*, 2 vols. (Oxford: Clarendon Press, 1964), vol. 1, p. 54.

22. Carleton B. Chapman, *Physicians, Law and Ethics* (New York: New York University Press, 1984), p. 71.

23. Clark, *A History of the Royal College*, vol. 1, pp. 208–217.

24. Clark, *A History of the Royal College*, vol. I, p. 95.

25. Chapman, *Physicians, Law and Ethics*, p. 66.

26. Clark, *A History of the Royal College*, vol. I, Appendix I, pp. 383–384. The ethical statutes also require attendance at college meetings unless ill or detained in prison.

27. Chapman, *Physicians, Law and Ethics*, p. 67.

28. In Europe, Joannes Siccus' *De Optimo Medico* (1551), Giovanni Codronchus' *De Christiana ac Tuta Medendi Ratione* (1591), Rodrigo à Castro's *Medicus Politicus* (1614), and Paulo Zacchias' *Quaestiones Medico-Legales* (1621–1635) and, in England, works by John Securis (1566) and John Cotta (1612).

29. Rodrigo à Castro, *Medicus Politicus sive De Officiis Medico-Politicis Tractatus, quatuor distinctis Libris: In quibus non solum Bonorum Medicorum mores ac virutes exprimuntur, malorum vero fraudes et imposturae deteguntur. Opus admodum utile medicis, aegrotis, aegrotorum assistentibus et cunctis aliis litterarum atque adeo politicae disciplinae cultoribus.* (Hamburg: Ex bibliopolio Frobeniano, 1614). Fielding H. Garrison and Leslie T. Morton, *A Medical Bibliography*, 3rd ed. (Philadelphia: J. B. Lippincott, 1970), p. 1759. On à Castro's life, see Schleiner, *Medical Ethics in the Renaissance*.

30. À Castro, *Medicus Politicus*, I, ii.

31. *Medicus Politicus*, III, ii.

32. *Medicus Politicus*, III, ix.

33. *Medicus Politicus*, III, ix–xxi.

34. Friedrich Hoffman, *Medicus Politicus, sive Regulae Prudentiae secundum quas medicus juvenis studia sua et vitae rationem dirigere debit si Famem sibi Felicemque Praxin et cito acquirere et conservare cupit* (Geneva: Fratres de Tournes, 1749), I, i.

35. *Medicus Politicus*, III, iii.

36. *Medicus Politicus*, III, iv.

37. Roger French, "Ethics in the Eighteenth Century: Hoffman at Halle," in Andrew Wear, Johanna Geyer-Kordesch, and Roger French (eds.), *Doctors and Ethics: The Earlier Historical Setting of Professional Ethics* (Amsterdam and Atlanta: Editions Rodopi B.V., 1993), pp. 153–180, quote on p. 175.

38. Johann Peter Frank, *System einer vollständigen medicinischen Polizei* (1779–1817), partially translated as *A System of Complete Medical Police*, Erna Lesky, trans. (Baltimore: Johns Hopkins University Press, 1976), pp. 391, 23, xvii. The term *Polizei* was used to designate a new science then appearing in the universities of Europe. That science, says Frank, concerns "the internal security of the State. . . . Medical police, like all police science, is an art of defense, a model of protection of people and their animal helpers against the deleterious consequences of dwelling together in large numbers, but especially of promoting their physical well-being so that people will succumb as late as possible to their eventual fate from the many physical illnesses to which they are subject." Introduction, p. 12. On Frank, see George Rosen, *From Medical Police to Social Medicine* (New York: Science History Publications, 1974), pp. 120–159.

39. Robert N. Proctor, *Racial Hygiene: Medicine Under the Nazis* (Cambridge: Harvard University Press, 1988).

40. Robert Nye, "Honor codes and medical ethics in modern France," *Bulletin of the History of Medicine* 69 (1995): 91–111, pp. 99, 104.

41. Geoffrey Chaucer, *Canterbury Tales*, ed. A. C. Cawley (London: Everyman's Library, 1958), Prologue, 411–444, pp. 13–14; François Rabelais, *Gargantua and Pantagruel*, trans. J. M. Cohen (London: Penguin Books, 1981) III, 32; Michel de Montaigne, *The Complete Essays of Montaigne*, trans. Donald M. Frame (Palo Alto: Stanford University Press, 1965), p. 581; Molière, *Malade Imaginaire*, III, iii; Molière, *L'Amour médecin*, II, v; Molière, *Monsieur de Pourceaugnac*, I, ii. *Oeuvres Complètes* (Paris: Editions du Seuil, 1962).

42. Cited in Francis Packard, *Guy Patin and the Medical Profession in Paris in the XVII Century* (New York: Augustus Kelly, 1970), p. 232.

43. Fynes Moryson, *Itinerary*, ed. Charles Hughes (Glasgow: J MacLehose, 1907), p. 424, cited in Carlo M. Cipolla, *Public Health and the Medical Profession in the Renaissance* (Cambridge: Cambridge University Press, 1976), p. 107.

5. British Medicine: Eighteenth and Nineteenth Centuries

1. Mary Fissel, "Innocent and honorable bribes: medical manners in eighteenth century Britain," in Robert Baker, Dorothy Porter, and Roy Porter (eds.), *The Codification of Medical Morality: Historical and Philosophical Studies of the Formalization of Western Medical Morality in the Eighteenth and Nineteenth Centuries* (Dordrect and Boston: Kluwer Academic Publishers, 1993); on the concept of gentleman, see Steven Shapin, *A Social History of Truth. Civility and Science in Seventeenth Century England* (Chicago: University of Chicago Press, 1994).

2. David Harley, "Honor and property: the structure of professional disputes in eighteenth-century England," in Andrew Cunningham and Roger French (eds.), *The Medical Enlightenment of the Eighteenth Century* (Cambridge: Cambridge University Press, 1990).

3. Adrian Wilson, "Politics of medical improvement," in Cunningham and French (eds.), *The Medical Enlightenment of the Eighteenth Century.*

4. George Eliot, *Middlemarch: A Study of Provincial Life*, ed. Bert Hornback (New York: W. W. Norton, 1977; first edition published by Chicago: Belford, Clarke, 1871).

5. John Pickstone, "Thomas Percival and the production of medical ethics," in Baker et al. (eds.), *The Codification of Medical Morality*.

6. Thomas Percival, *Medical Ethics; or, a Code of Institutes and Precepts, Adapted to the Professional Conduct of Physicians and Surgeons* (London: S. Russell, 1803). The modern edition is *Percival's Medical Ethics*, ed. Chauncey Leake (Baltimore: Williams & Wilkins, 1927).

7. Justinian. *Institutes* I; Percival, Preface, in Leake (ed.), *Percival's Medical Ethics*, p. 69.

8. Percival, Preface, in Leake (ed.), *Percival's Medical Ethics*, p. 67.

9. Percival, Preface, in Leake (ed.), *Percival's Medical Ethics*, p. 65.

10. Percival, Dedication, in Leake (ed.), *Percival's Medical Ethics*, p. 63.

11. Percival, ch. I, 1, in Leake (ed.), *Percival's Medical Ethics*, p. 71.

12. Percival, ch. II, 32, in Leake (ed.), *Percival's Medical Ethics*, p. 111.

13. Percival, Preface, in Leake (ed.), *Percival's Medical Ethics*, p. 68; Roy Porter, "Thomas Gisborne: Physicians, Christians and gentlemen," in Wear et al. (eds.), *Doctors and Ethics*, pp. 252–273.

14. Percival, "Notes and Illustrations," in Leake (ed.), p. 187; James Boswell, *Life of Johnson* (London: Henry Frowde, 1904), vol. II, p. 559. Ironically, exactly six months after making this remark, Johnson was on his deathbed. He asked his physician, Dr. Brockelsby, "a man in whom he had confidence, to tell him plainly whether he could recover. 'Give me [said he] a direct answer." On being given the direct answer he sought ["not without a miracle"], Johnson said, "I will take no more physick, not even my opiates, for I have prayed that I may render up my soul to God unclouded." *Life*, vol. II, p. 644.

15. Percival, "Notes and Illustrations," in Leake (ed.), *Percival's Medical Ethics*, pp. 187, 188, 191, 194, 193; Robert Baker, "Disciphering Percival's code," in Baker et al. (eds.),*The Codification of Medical Morality*; Thomas Gisborne, *An Enquiry into the Duties of Men in the Higher and Middle Classes of Society in Great Britain*, 2 vols., 2nd ed. (London: B. & J. White, 1795).

16. John Gregory, *Observations on the Duties and Offices of a Physician and on the Method of Promoting Enquiry in Philosophy* (London: Strahan and Cadell, 1770), p. 11. This is an edition of Gregory's lectures based on the lecture notes of Gregory's students in 1770 and possibly redacted by his son, James. Gregory corrected and expanded the next edition, titled *Lectures on the Duties and Offices of a Physician*, which was published in 1772. The modern edition of both works is Lawrence McCullough (ed)., *John Gregory's Writings on Medical Ethics and Philosophy of Medicine* (Dordrecht: Kluwer Academic Press, 1997). John's son, James Gregory, also contributed to the literature in medical ethics rather differently than did his father. His *Memorial to the Managers of the Royal Infirmary* (1800) exposed the abuses of the public hospital in Edinburgh and, in so doing, developed a full set of rights for patients, derived from the physician's primary duty to help the sick and not expose them to danger. James' criticism of the practices of his colleagues won him nothing but disdain and anger. Another Edinburgh practitioner, John Bell, felt compelled to "chastise this rude and blundering physician" in a massive tome entitled, *Letters on the Professional Character and Manners Addressed to James Gregory* (Edinburgh: John Moir, 1810), p. vii.

17. Gregory, *Lectures*, p. 19.

18. Robert Baker, "The History of Medical Ethics," in W. F. Bynum and Roy Porter (eds.), *Companion Encyclopedia of the History of Medicine*, 2 vols. (London and New

York: Routledge, 1993). vol. 2, p. 861; Laurence B. McCullough, who has recently edited Gregory's works, has also written an extensive biography, arguing for his place in the history of modern medical ethics *John Gregory and the Invention of Professional Medical Ethics and the Profession of Medicine* (Dordrecht and Boston: Kluwer Academic Publishers, 1998); see also McCullough, "John Gregory (1724–1773) and the invention of professional relationships in medicine," *Journal of Clinical Ethics* 8 (Spring 1997): 11–21; McCullough, "Historical perspectives on the ethical dimensions of the physician–patient relationship: the medical ethics of Dr. John Gregory," *Ethics in Science and Medicine* 5 (1978): 47–53; McCullough, "Virtues, etiquette and Anglo-American medical ethics in the eighteenth century," in Earl E. Shelp (ed.), *Virtue and Medicine: Explorations into the Character of Medicine* (Dordrecht: Kluwer Academic Publishers, 1985); McCullough, "John Gregory's medical ethics and Humean sympathy," in Baker et al. (eds.), *The Codification of Medical Morality*. See also Tom L. Beauchamp, "Common sense and virtue in the Scottish philosophers," in Baker et al. (eds.), *The Codification of Medical Morality*.

19. Samuel Johnson, "On the death of Mr. Robert Levet, A Practiser in Physic," in Helen Gardner (ed.), *The New Book of Oxford English Verse 1250–1950* (Oxford: Oxford University Press, 1972), p. 436. The elegy appeared in *The Gentleman's Companion* in August 1783. At that time, *officious* meant "dedicated to duty." On Levit, see John Wain, *Samuel Johnson* (New York, Viking Press, 1974), passim.

20. Eliot, *Middlemarch*, p. 99.

21. On the debate over gynecological surgery, see Ann Dally, *Women Under the Knife. A History of Surgery* (London: Hutchinson Radius, 1991). One debate that spread outside the profession's control was the vigorous discussion of vivisection, the experimental use of animals. See Richard D. French, *Antivivisection and Medical Science in Victorian Society* (Princeton: Princeton University Press, 1975) and James Turner, *Reckoning with the Beast. Animals, Pain and Humanity in the Victorian Mind* (Baltimore: Johns Hopkins University Press, 1980).

22. Roy Porter, "Medical ethics, history of nineteenth-century Great Britain," in Reich (ed.), *Encyclopedia of Bioethics*, vol. III, p. 1553.

6. Ethics in American Medicine

1. Two useful histories of American medicine are John S. Haller, Jr., *American Medicine in Transition 1840–1910* (Urbana: University of Illinois Press, 1981), and William G. Rothstein, *American Physicians in the Nineteenth Century: From Sects to Science* (Baltimore: Johns Hopkins University Press, 1972).

2. Genevieve Miller, *The Adoption of Inoculation for smallpox in England and France* (Philadelphia: University of Pennsylvania Press, 1957); Adrian Wilson, "Politics of medical improvement," in Cunningham and French (eds.), *The Medical Enlightenment of the Eighteenth Century*.

3. Cotton Mather, "Variolae triumphatae," in *The Angel of Bethesda*, ed. Gordon W. Jones (reprint, Barre, Mass.: Barre Publishers, 1972), pp. 93–116, section on inoculation, pp. 107–116.

4. Samuel Bard, "Discourse on the Duties of a Physician with some Sentiments on the Usefulness and Necessity of a Public Hospital" (King's College Commencement, May 16, 1769), published as *Advice to those Gentlemen Who Receive the First Medical Degree Conferred by that University* (New York: Robertson, 1769), pp. 2–3, 14, 6.

5. Carl Binger, *Revolutionary Doctor: Benjamin Rush, 1746–1813* (New York: W. W. Norton, 1966). See also Daniel J. Boorstin, *The Lost World of Thomas Jefferson* (New York: H. Holt, 1948), Ch. 3.

6. Benjamin Rush, *Inquiry into the Causes of Animal Life*, p. 40; *Inquiry into the Natural History of Medicine Among the Indians of North America*, p. 90; *Duties*, p. 264, in *Medical Inquiries and Observations* (New York: The Arno Press, 1972). Vol. 1.

7. Rush, Lecture V, "On virtues and vices of physicians," in *Six Introductory Lectures to the Course of Lectures upon the Institutes and Practice of Medicine* (Philadelphia: J. Conrad, 1801), pp. 121–142.

8. Rush, Lecture X, "On the means of acquiring business in the profession of medicine," in *Sixteen Introductory Lectures* (Philadelphia: Bradford and Innskeep, 1811), the second, expanded edition of *Six Introductory Lectures*.

9. Rush, Lecture X, "Observations on the duties of a physician and the methods of improving medicine," in *Sixteen Lectures*, pp. 256, 258, 260.

10. Rush, Lecture XIV, "On the duty of patients to their physicians," in *Sixteen Lectures*, pp. 319–339.

11. Robert Baker, "An introduction to the Boston medical police of 1808," in Robert Baker (ed.), *The Codification of Medical Morality: Historical and Philosophical Studies of the Formalization of Western Medical Morality in the Eighteenth and Nineteenth Centuries*, vol. 2 (Dordrecht and Boston: Kluwer Academic Publishers, 1995), pp. 25–40. On the formation of the medical profession in the United States, see Richard H. Shryock's two books: *Medicine and Society in America: 1660–1860* (Ithaca: Cornell University Press, 1960) and *Medical Licensing in America, 1650–1965* (Baltimore: Johns Hopkins University Press, 1967). See also Joseph F. Kett, *The Formation of the American Medical Profession. The Role of Institutions, 1780–1860* (New Haven: Yale University Press, 1968).

12. Chauncey D. Leake, "What was Kappa Lambda?" *Annals of Medical History* 4 (1922): 192–206; Francis R. Packard, *The History of Medicine in the United States* (New York: Hafner Publishing Co., 1963), vol. I, p. 478.

13. Richard H. Shryock, *Medicine in America* (Baltimore: Johns Hopkins University Press, 1966), pp. 150–151, quoting the *Philadelphia City Item*, Nov. 6, 1858, and *Cincinnati Medical Observer* 2 (1857): 129. John Duffy, *The Healers. A History of American Medicine* (Urbana: University of Illinois Press, 1979), pp. 180–186. *Proceeding of the Physico-Medical Society of New Orleans* (New Orleans, 1838), pp. 24–25.

14. Dr. Charles Devol's Case Book is a manuscript in the library of the Department of Medical History and Ethics, University of Washington School of Medicine, a gift of James Haviland, M.D. Dr. Haviland had it from a descendant of the writer. Dr. James Whorton, Professor of Medical History at the University of Washington, believes, on the basis of Devol's manner of practice, that his casebook dates from the late 1840s or early 1850s. The essay on ethics may have been copied from some unknown source, but I judge it to be his personal reflections. The Case Book is not paginated.

15. Haller, *American Medicine in Transition*, p. 118.

16. Norman Gevitz (ed.), *Other Healers. Unorthodox Medicine in America* (Baltimore: Johns Hopkins University Press, 1988).

17. American Medical Association, "Code of Ethics 1847," in Leake (ed.), *Percival's Medical Ethics*, p. 222.

18. John Bell, "Introduction to the Code of Medical Ethics," in Baker et al. (eds.), *The Codification of Medical Morality*, vol. 2, pp. 65–72, quote on pp. 65, 66.

19. Robert Baker, "The historical context of the American Medical Association's 1847

Code of Ethics," in Baker et al. (eds.), *The Codification of Medical Ethics*, vol. 2, pp. 47–64. I owe to Baker's essay my exegesis of the first draft of The Code.

20. Code of Ethics, 1847, Chapter II, iv, in Leake (ed.), *Percival's Medical Ethics*, pp. 228–229.

21. Haller, *American Medicine in Transition*, p. 237.

22. Francis Delafield, "Presidential Address to the Association of American Physicians," *Journal of the American Medical Association* 7 (1886): 16.

23. James G. Burrow, *AMA: Voice of American Medicine* (Baltimore: Johns Hopkins University Press, 1963); Donald Konold, *A History of American Medical Ethics, 1847–1912* (Madison: State Historical Society of Wisconsin, 1962).

24. George Wood, "Editorial," *Transactions of the AMA* 9 (1856): 61.

25. Austin Flint, *Medical Ethics and Etiquette: The National Code of Medical Ethics* (New York: D. Appleton and Company, 1883); Nathan Smith Davis, *History of Medicine, with the Code of Medical Ethics* (Chicago: Cleveland Press, 1907).

26. Nathan Smith Davis, "Editorial," *Journal of the American Medical Association* 1 (1883): 57.

27. The Committee on Medical Ethics of State Medical Society of Ohio, published as M. B. Wright, "Report of the Special Committee on Medical Ethics," *Transactions of the Ohio State Medical Society* (1855): 37.

28. Alfred Carroll and John C. Peters, "Code of Ethics," *Medical Gazette of New York* 3 (1869): 150. Ironically, this criticism anticipates a twentieth-century interpretation of the Code, which sees it entirely as an instrument to attain a medical monopoly, without any distinguishing moral characteristics. See Jeffery L. Berlant, *Profession and Monopoly: A Study of Medicine in the United States and Great Britain* (Berkeley: University of California Press, 1975). See Robert Baker, Dorothy Porter, and Roy Porter, "Introduction," in Baker et al. (eds.), *The Codification of Medical Morality*, vol. 1, pp. 1–15. For the refutation of this position, see Baker, "Introduction," in Baker et al. (eds.), *The Codification of Medical Morality*, vol. 2, pp. 1–24; Kett, *The Formation of the American Medical Profession*, p. 176.

29. Worthington Hooker, *Physician and Patient, or a Practical View of the Mutual Duties, Relations and Interests of the Medical Profession and the Community* (New York: Baker and Scribner, 1849), reprint ed. (New York: Arno Press, Inc., 1972).

30. Hooker, *Physician and Patient*, pp. 257–258.

31. Chapter I, "Uncertainty of medicine"; Chapter II, "Skill in medicine"; Chapter III, "Popular errors." See also Hooker, *History of Medical Delusions* (New York: Baker and Scribner, 1850), pp. 7–8, 33; Tom L. Beauchamp, "Worthington Hooker on ethics in clinical medicine," in Baker et al. (eds.), *The Codification of Medical Morality*, vol. 2, pp. 105–119.

32. Flint, *Medical Ethics and Etiquette*, pp. 1–4.

33. Rosemary Stevens, *American Medicine and the Public Interest* (New Haven: Yale University Press, 1971).

34. Herbert M. Morais, *The History of the Negro in Medicine* (New York: Association for the Study of Negro Life and History, 1967), pp. 54–58.

35. Regina Morantz-Sanchez, *Sympathy and Science* (New York: Oxford University Press, 1985), p. 183. See also Ellen Singer More and Maureen A. Milligan, *The Empathic Practitioner: Empathy, Gender and Medicine* (New Brunswick, N.J.: Rutgers University Press, 1994; Ellen More, *Restoring the Balance: Women Physicians and the Profession of Medicine* (Cambridge: Harvard University Press, 1999).

36. Marc A. Rodwin, *Medicine, Money, and Morals: Physicians' Conflicts of Interest* (New York: Oxford University Press, 1993); Loyal Davis, *Fellowship of Surgeons: History of the American College of Surgeons* (Springfield: Charles C. Thomas, 1960).

37. James Gordon Burrow, *AMA: Voice of American Medicine* (Baltimore: Johns Hopkins University Press, 1963); Burrow, *Organized Medicine in the Progressive Era: The Move Toward Monopoly* (Baltimore: Johns Hopkins University Press, 1977).

38. Haller, *American Medicine in Transition*, p. 283.

39. Benjamin Rush, "On the influence of physical causes on the moral faculty," delivered before the American Philosophical Society, February 27, 1786, reprinted in Dagobert D. Runes (ed.), *The Selected Writings of Benjamin Rush* (New York: Philosophical Library, 1947), pp. 181–211.

40. Bell, "Introduction to the Code of Medical Ethics," in Baker et al. (eds.), *The Codification of Medical Morality*, vol. 2, p. 68.

41. Hooker, *Physician and Patient*, p. 391.

42. John S. Haller, Jr., and Robin Haller, *The Physician and Sexuality in Victorian America* (Urbana: University of Illinois Press, 1974), pp. 148–163.

43. James C. Whorton, *Crusaders for Fitness: The History of American Health Reformers* (Princeton: Princeton University Press, 1982), p. 111.

44. Charles C. Rosenberg, *No Other Gods. On Science and American Social Thought* (Baltimore: Johns Hopkins University Press, 1976), pp. 10–11; Haller and Haller, *The Physician and Sexuality in Victorian America;* Whorton, *Crusaders for Fitness*; Robert M. Veatch, "Diverging traditions: professional and religious medical ethics of the nineteenth century," in Baker et al. (eds.), *The Codification of Medical Morality*, vol. 2, pp. 121–135. American physicians were not all "moralistic": many took serious interest in social reform and civil rights. See Eugene Perry Link, *The Social Ideas of American Physicians (1776–1976)* (London and Toronto: Associated University Presses, 1992).

45. Woods Hutchinson, *The Gospel According to Darwin* (Chicago: Open Court Press, 1898); see Whorton, *Crusaders for Fitness*.

46. *AMA Code of 1847*, Chapter I, articles I and vii, in Leake (ed.), *Percival's Medical Ethics*, p. 221.

47. G. Morant, *Hints to Husbands: A Revelation of the Man-Midwife Mysteries* (London, 1857), p. 7; Haller, *American Medicine in Transition*, p. 155.

48. William P. Dewees, "Compendious system of midwifery, chiefly designed to facilitate the inquires of those who may be pursuing this branch of study," *Philosophy* (1824): 190–191. See Edward A. Shorter, *A History of Women's Bodies* (New York: Basic Books, 1982); Judith W. Leavitt, *Brought to Bed. Childbearing in America 1750–1850* (New York: Oxford University Press, 1986).

49. *Public Statute Laws of the State of Connecticut, Crimes and Punishments*, 1821, section 14; James C. Mohr, *Abortion in America: The Origins and Evolution of National Policy 1800–1900* (New York: Oxford University Press, 1978), p. 21.

50. *Revised Statutes of New York.* 1828–1835, I, Title VI, Ch. I, Part IV, section 21; Mohr, *Abortion in America*, p. 27.

51. "Report on Criminal Abortion," *Transactions of the American Medical Association*, XII (1859), 75–78; Mohr, *Abortion in America*, p. 157.

52. Mohr, *Abortion in America*, p. 157.

53. John Todd, *Serpents in the Doves' Nest* (Boston: 1867), p. 6; Mohr, *Abortion in America*, p. 187.

54. Mohr, *Abortion in America*, p. 301. Mohr incorrectly states that, in 1869, the Church reiterated its medieval condemnation of abortion; in fact, it repudiated the medieval form of that condemnation. The 1869 statement of Pope Pius IX abolished the distinction between the abortion of an "animated fetus" and an "unanimated fetus," which allowed that a serious reason could justify abortion of the latter; the pope applied the penalty of excommunication to both. The history of the Roman Catholic Church's position on abortion

is more complex than is usually presented. After centuries during which the abortion of an unanimated fetus was judged less sinful than the abortion of an animated one and the desperate saving of the mother's life by abortion was tolerated, the Church moved to a more rigorous position in the eighteenth century, declaring that fetal life from conception must be protected and that no direct abortion, for whatever reason, could be tolerated. A theological disagreement over the permissibility of *craniotomy* (a procedure similar to that now called *partial birth abortion*) to save the mother's life was decided in the negative by Vatican decrees in 1884, 1889, and 1895. However, Catholic doctors were permitted to perform an *indirect abortion* in which fetal life was terminated when a maternal pathology, such as a cancerous uterus, was removed. See John R. Connery, *Abortion. The Development of the Roman Catholic Perspective* (Chicago: Loyola University Press, 1977).

55. Mohr, *Abortion in America*, pp. 6, 166.

7. American Medicine: Science, Competence, and Ethics

1. *Code of Ethics*, 1847, Chapter II, article iv, in Leake (ed.), *Percival's Medical Ethics*, pp. 228–229.

2. Charles Singer and A. Ashworth Underwood, *A Short History of Medicine* (New York: Oxford University Press, 1962), p. 236.

3. Martin S. Pernick, *A Calculus of Suffering. Pain, Professionalism and Anesthesia in Nineteenth-Century America* (New York: Columbia University Press, 1985).

4. William Sargent, n.t., *American Journal of Medicine and Science* 23 (1852): 455; Pernick, *Calculus of Suffering*, p. 91.

5. *Transactions of the AMA* 1848, I: 189–196; Pernick, *Calculus of Suffering*, p. 37.

6. *Philadelphial Medical Examiner* 3 (October 1847): 635; Pernick, *Calculus of Suffering*, p. 62.

7. Pernick, *Calculus of Suffering*, p. 79.

8. Pernick, *Calculus of Suffering*, p. 95.

9. *Transactions of the AMA* 1 (1848):176; Pernick, *Calculus of Suffering*, p. 94.

10. Hooker, *Physician and Patient*, p. 56; Pernick, *Calculus of Suffering*, p. 100.

11. Pernick, *Calculus of Suffering*, pp. 101–102.

12. Daniel Fox, "The segregation of medical ethics: a problem in modern intellectual history," *Journal of Medicine and Philosophy* 4, no. 1 (1974): 81–94.

13. James did discuss animal experimentation and the licensing of physicians but only as passing comments on events of the time. See Gerald E. Myers, *William James: His Life and Thought* (New Haven: Yale University Press, 1986).

14. Bell, "Introduction to the Code of Medical Ethics," in Baker et al. (eds.), *The Codification of Medical Morality*, vol. 2, p. 66; Francis Wayland, *The Elements of Moral Science II: Duties Toward Man*, (Boston: Gould and Lincoln, 1854) pp. 190–196; Chester Burns, "Reciprocity in the development of Anglo-American medical ethics, 1765–1865," in Baker et al. (eds.), *The Codification of Medical Morality*, vol. 2, pp. 135–144.

15. Baker, "Historical context of the American Medical Association's 1847 *Code of Ethics*," in Baker et al. (eds.), *The Codification of Medical Morality*, vol. 2, pp. 47–64.

16. Fox, "Segregation of medical ethics," p. 83.

17. Bell, "Introduction to the Code of Medical Ethics," in Baker et al. (eds.), *The Codification of Medical Morality*, vol. 2, p. 65.

18. Thomas H. Huxley, *Collected Essays, 1893–1894* (Hildesheim and New York: George Alms Verlag, 1970), vol. 3, cited in Fox, "Segregation of medical ethics," p. 87.

19. Richard C. Cabot, *Case Histories in Medicine* (Boston: W. M. Leonard, 1911).

20. Richard C. Cabot, *Social Work: Essays on the Meeting Ground of Doctor and Social Worker* (Boston and New York: Houghton Mifflin Company, 1919).

21. Richard C. Cabot, *The Meaning of Right and Wrong* (New York: Macmillan Company, 1933), pp. 13, 110. Cabot also produced another general treatise on moral philosophy, *What Men Live By* (Boston and New York: Houghton Mifflin Company, 1914).

22. Richard C. Cabot, *The Christian Approach to Social Morality* (New York: National Board of Young Women's Christian Association, 1913); Cabot and Russell L. Dicks, *The Art of Ministering to the Sick* (New York: The Macmillan Company, 1936).

23. Chester Burns, "Richard Cabot and reformation in American medical ethics," *Bulletin of the History of Medicine* 51 (1977): 353–368, quote on p. 368.

24. *Nosokomeion* 2 (1931): 151–161.

25. Albert R. Jonsen, *The New Medicine and the Old Ethics* (Cambridge and London: Harvard University Press, 1990), p. 27.

26. Burns, "Richard Cabot," pp. 358–359; Cabot, "A study of mistaken diagnosis," *Journal of the American Medical Association* 55 (1910): 1343–1350; Cabot, "Diagnostic pitfalls identified during a study of three thousand autopsies," *Journal of the American Medical Association* 59 (1912): 2295–2298.

27. Francis W. Peabody, "The care of the patient," *Journal of the American Medical Association* 88 (1927): 877–881, p. 881.

28. Cabot, *What Men Live By* (Boston: Houghton Mifflin, 1914), pp. xi, xii.

29. Cabot, *Training and Rewards of the Physician* (Philadelphia: J. B. Lippincott Company, 1918).

30. Cabot, *Training and Rewards of the Physician*, p. 52.

31. Cabot, *Training and Rewards of the Physician*, p. 151.

32. Cabot, Preface, in *Honesty* (New York: Macmillan Company, 1938).

33. Cabot, "Truth and falsity in medicine," *American Medicine* 5 (1903): 344–349, p. 344; Cabot, *Honesty*; Cabot, *Ethical Forces in the Practice of Medicine* (Cambridge: Harvard University Press, 1905).

34. Cabot, "Truth and falsity," p. 344.

35. Joseph Collins, "Should doctors tell the truth?" *Harper's Monthly Magazine* 155 (1927): 320–326, quote on p. 322.

36. The first rigorous experimental study of this contentious moral matter did not appear until 1961. Dr. Donald Oken designed a survey questionnaire to determine the attitudes of physicians toward truth-telling and the rationales for those attitudes. He was able to show that some 90 percent of physicians frequently withheld a diagnosis of cancer from their patients, offering as the rationale the importance of encouraging hope and discouraging depression and suicide. He was also able to show that few physicians had much information about whether their policy of dissembling actually had the desired results. Donald Oken, "What to tell cancer patients," *Journal of the American Medical Association* 175 (1961): 1120–1128.

37. Cabot, *Adventures on the Borderlands of Ethics* (New York: Harper and Brothers, 1926).

38. On Cabot's influence, see Ida Maud Cannon, *On the Social Frontier of Medicine: Pioneering in Medical Social Service* (Cambridge: Harvard University Press, 1952); T. F. Williams, "Cabot, Peabody and the care of the patient," *Bulletin of the History of Medicine* 24 (1950): 462–481; Burns, "Richard Cabot."

39. Robert B. Bean and William B. Bean (eds.), William Osler, *Aphorisms from His Bedside Teachings and Writings*, (Springfield: Charles C. Thomas, 1951), p. 88. Osler

remarks in a footnote on the ethics of medical experimentation in terms that anticipate modern views: *Principles and Practice of Medicine*, 3rd ed. (New York: Appleton, 1898), p. 18.

40. William Osler, *Aequanimitas: Valedictory Remarks to the Graduates in Medicine of the University of Pennsylvania, May 1, 1889* (Philadelphia: W. F. Fell and Company, 1889); *Aequanamitas, with Other Addresses to Medical Students, Nurses and Practitioners of Medicine* (Philadelphia: P. Blakiston's Son, 1904), p. 4.

41. Harvey Cushing, *The Life of Sir William Osler*, vol. II (Oxford: at the Clarendon Press, 1925), p. 685; William Osler, "Chauvinism in Medicine," *Montreal Medical Journal* 31 (1902): 684, cited in Bean and Bean (eds.), *Sir William Osler*, p. 118.

42. See Susan Lederer, *Subjected to Science:Human Experimentation in America before the Second World War* (Baltimore: Johns Hopkins University Press, 1995); Jonsen, *The Birth of Bioethics*, ch. 5. The citation from Claude Bernard is from *Introduction to the Study of Experimental Medicine*, trans. H. Greene (New York: Dover Books, 1957), ch. II, sec. iii, pp. 101–102.

43. Paul Ramsey, *The Patient as Person: Explorations in Medical Ethics* (New Haven: Yale University Press, 1970), p. xv.

44. Chauncey D. Leake, "Theories of ethics and human experimentation," *Annals of the New York Academy of Science* 169 (1970): 388–396; Leake, "The interesting case of Furan aspirin," *Texas Reports on Biology and Medicine* 30, no. 2 (1972): 105–107.

45. Chauncey D. Leake, *The Old Egyptian Medical Papyri* (Lawrence: University of Kansas Press, 1952).

46. Chauncey Leake and Patrick Romanell, *Can We Agree? A Scientist and a Philosopher Argue About Ethics* (Austin: University of Texas Press, 1950). The articles collected in this book appeared as Leake, "Ethicogenesis," *Scientific Monthly* 60 (1945): 245–253 (originally delivered at the 1940 American Association for the Advancement of Science Symposium on Science and Ethics) and P. Romanell "Reply to Ethicogenesis," *Scientific Monthly* 61 (1945): 293–306; Leake, "A scientific versus a metaphysical approach to ethics," *Scientific Monthly* 62 (1946): 187–92.

47. Leake (ed.), *Percival's Medical Ethics*, p. 5; Warner Fite, *An Introductory Study of Ethics* (New York: Longmans, Green, 1916).

48. Leake (ed.), *Percival's Medical Ethics*.

49. W. H. S. Jones, *The Doctor's Oath: An Essay in the History of Medicine* (Cambridge: Cambridge University Press, 1924); see Leake (ed.), *Percival's Medical Ethics*, p. 18. Recall that Austin Flint's 1883 commentary on the AMA Code was titled *Medical Ethics and Etiquette*; Gregory and others also suggest the distinction.

50. Leake (ed.), *Percival's Medical Ethics*, p. xxix.

51. See Baker, Introduction, in Baker et al. (eds.), *The Codification of Medical Morality*, vol. 2, pp. 3–6.

52. Leake, "How is medical ethics to be taught?" *Bulletin of the Association of American Medical Colleges* 3 (1928): 341–343.

53. Leake, *What Are We Living For?: A Practical Philosophy* (Westbury, New York: PJD Publications, 1973).

54. The story of the Cartesian illumination is told in Leake, " A scientific vs. a metaphysical approach to ethics," *Scientific Monthly* 62 (1941): 187–192, and also in J. Herrick, "Little academies I have known," *Scientific Monthly* 53 (1941): 133. Some years later, Leake acknowledged that he found the work of Joseph Fletcher, particularly *Situation Ethics* (Philadelphia: Westminster Press, 1966), "a most satisfactory representation of his own thought." Leake, Preface to the Second Edition of *Percival's Medical Ethics*, p. li.

55. Leake (ed.), *Percival's Medical Ethics*, p. xxxii.

56. Leake, "How is medical ethics to be taught?" p. 343.

57. Cabot and Dicks, *The Art of Ministering to the Sick* (New York: The Macmillan Co., 1936). Catholic doctors had long contributed to "pastoral medicine"; see Austin O'Malley and James J. Walsh, *Essays in Pastoral Medicine* (New York: Longmans, Green, 1906); Austin O'Malley, *The Ethics of Medical Homicide and Mutilation* (New York: Devin-Adair, 1919).

58. Charles Coppens, *Moral Principles and Medical Practice: The Basis of American Jurisprudence* (New York: Benziger Brothers, 1897); Gerald P. Kelly, *Medico-Moral Problems*, 5 parts (St. Louis: The Catholic Hospital Association of the United States, 1949–1954). The history of Catholic moral theology's interest in medical ethics is found in Kelly, *The Emergence of Roman Catholic Medical Ethics in North America: A Historical-Methodological-Biographical Study*. Most rabbinical studies of medico-moral issues appeared in Hebrew until the major work of Rabbi Immanuel Jakobovits, *Jewish Medical Ethics. A Comparative and Historical Study of the Jewish Religious Attitude to Medicine and Its Practice* (New York: Bloch, 1959).

59. George Jacoby, *Physician, Pastor and Patient. Problems in Pastoral Medicine* (New York: P. B. Hoeber, Inc. 1936).

60. Willard L. Sperry, *Ethical Basis of Medical Care* (New York: P. B. Hoeber, Inc. 1950).

61. Harold Vanderpool, "What medical ethics used to look like" (paper presented at the Birth of Bioethics Conference, Seattle, September 23–24, 1992), transcript pp. 376–378.

62. Joseph Fletcher, *Morals and Medicine* (Boston: Beacon Press, 1954), p. 25.

63. On Fletcher, see Albert R. Jonsen, *The Birth of Bioethics* (New York: Oxford University Press, 1998); Kenneth Vaux (ed.), *Memoir of an Ex-Radical: Reminscence and Reappraisal* (Louisville: Westminster/John Knox Press, 1993).

64. Personal communication from James Whorton to Albert Jonsen.

65. *Code of Ethics*, 1847, III, art. 1, 3; 1903, II, art. iv, 1, in Leake (ed.), *Percival's Medical Ethics*, pp. 235, 254.

66. *Principles of Medical Ethics*, 1912, II, art. 6, 1, in Leake (ed.), *Percival's Medical Ethics*, p. 270.

67. *Principles of Medical Ethics*, 1957, in Leake (ed.), *Percival's Medical Ethics*, p. 278.

68. American Medical Association, *Code of Medical Ethics* (Chicago: AMA, 1997), xi.

69. Cabot, *Training and Rewards*, pp. 133, 136.

70. The most detailed analysis of this professional progress is Paul Starr, *The Social Transformation of American Medicine* (New York: Basic Books, 1982).

71. Estelle Raben, "*Men in White* and *Yellow Jack* as mirrors of the medical profession," *Literature and Medicine* 12 (1993): 19–41, p. 20.

72. Chester R. Burns, "Fictional doctors and the evolution of medical ethics in the United States, 1875–1900," *Literature and Medicine* 7 (1988): 39–55; Richard Malmsheimer, *"Doctors Only." The Evolving Image of the American Physician* (New York: Greenwood Press, 1988). Medical writers since ancient times have asserted that the demeanor of the kindly doctor benefits his or her patients, improving their compliance with treatment and evoking the placebo effect that makes sick persons better even if their medicine fails. However, little scientific evidence exists in proof of this assertion. In recent years, some professional groups have become interested in defining and evalu-

ating the "humanistic qualities" of physicians and in measuring the outcomes of these qualities on the well-being of patients. See, for example, American Board of Internal Medicine, *Project Professionalism* (Philadelphia: American Board of Internal Medicine, 1989).

8. A Chronicle of Ethical Events: 1940s to 1980s

1. G. E. W. Wolstenholme (ed.), *Man and His Future* (Boston: Little, Brown and Company, 1963), n.p. This volume is the proceedings of a conference sponsored by Ciba Foundation in 1962.

2. Albert R. Jonsen, *The Birth of Bioethics* (New York: Oxford University Press, 1998).

3. *Trials of War Criminals before the Nuremberg Military Tribunals* (Washington, D.C.: U.S. Government Printing Office, 1949), vol. 2, p. 181; Jonsen, *The Birth of Bioethics*, ch. 5.

4. Eva Moses-Kor, "The Mengele twins and human experimentation: a personal account," in George J. Annas and Michael A. Grodin (eds.), *The Nazi Doctors and the Nuremberg Code: Human Rights in Human Experimentation* (New York: Oxford University Press, 1992); Telford Taylor, "The opening statement of the prosecution, Dec. 9, 1946," in *The Nazi Doctors and the Nuremberg Code*; see Gerald L. Poser and John Ware; *Mengele: The Complete Story* (New York: McGraw-Hill, 1986); Lucette Matalon Lagnado and Sheila Cohn Dekel, *Children of the Flames: The Untold Story of the Twins of Auschwitz* (New York: William Morrow, 1991); Robert J. Lifton, *The Nazi Doctors: Medical Killing and the Psychology of Genocide* (New York: Basic Books, 1986); Alexander Mitscherlich and Fred Mielke, *Doctors of Infamy: The Story of the Nazi Medical Crimes* (New York: H. Schuman, 1949).

5. "Report on war crimes of a medical nature committed in Germany and elsewhere on German nationals and the nationals of occupied countries by the Nazi Regime during World War II," *AMA Archives*, quoted from Advisory Committee on Human Radiation Experiments, *Final Report* (Washington, D.C.: U.S. Government Printing Office, 1995), pp. 133–134. The most compelling commentary on the Nazi medical crimes was written by another American physician closely associated with the trial, Leo Alexander, "Medical science under dictatorship," *New England Journal of Medicine* 241 (1949): 39–47, quote on p. 44; see also Annas and Grodin, *The Nazi Doctors and the Nuremberg Code*; Arthur L. Caplan (ed.), *When Medicine Went Mad: Bioethics and the Holocaust* (Totawa, N.J.: Humana Press, 1952).

6. James Watson and Francis Crick, "The molecular structure of nucleic acids," *Nature* 4356 (April 25, 1953): 737; Jonsen, *The Birth of Bioethics*, ch. 6.

7. "Clue to chemistry of heredity found," *New York Times* (June 13, 1953), p. 17.

8. J. P. Merrill, J. E. Murray, J. H. Harrison, and W. R. Guild, "Successful homotransplantation of the human kidney between identical twins," *Journal of the American Medical Association* 160 (1956): 277–282; Jonsen, *The Birth of Bioethics*, ch. 7.

9. E. C. Padgett, "Is iso-skin grafting practicable?" *Southern Medical Journal* 25 (1932): 895; J. B. Brown, "Homografting of skin: with report of success in identical twins," *Surgery* 1 (1937): 558.

10. Paul Vaughn, *The Pill on Trial* (London: Weidenfeld and Nicholson, 1970), p. 47; on the broad moral questions, see Daniel Callahan (ed.), *The Catholic Case for Contraception* (New York: Macmillan Company, 1969); Jonsen, *The Birth of Bioethics*, ch. 9.

11. Shana Alexander, "They decide who lives, who dies," *Life* 53 (1962): 102–125; Jhan Robbins and June Robbins, "The rest are simply left to die," *Redbook* (November 1967): 80–81; an NBC Documentary, "Who Lives? Who Dies?" aired in 1965; Jonsen, *The Birth of Bioethics*, ch. 7.

12. David Saunders and Jesse Dukeminier, Jr., "Medical advance and legal lag: hemodialysis and kidney transplantation," *UCLA Law Review* 15 (1968): 366–380, quote on p. 378.

13. Nicholas Rescher, "The allocation of exotic life saving therapy," *Ethics* 79 (1969): 173–186; Samuel Gorovitz, "Ethics and the allocation of medical resources," *Medical Research Engineering* 5, no. 4 (1966): 5–7; Ramsey, *The Patient as Person*, (New Haven: Yale University Press, 1970), chapter 7; James Childress, "Who shall live when not all can live?" *Soundings* 53 (1970): 339–355. Renée C. Fox and Judith P. Swazey, *The Courage to Fail: A Social View of Organ Transplant and Dialysis* (Chicago: Chicago University Press, 1974), tells the full story of the Seattle Artificial Kidney Center and its selection program. The committee was never officially terminated, but it ceased to meet after Congress passed the End-Stage Renal Disease Amendments in 1973, providing financial support for patients in need of renal dialysis and transplantation.

14. "The ultimate operation," *Time* (December 15, 1967): 64–72; Jonsen, *The Birth of Bioethics*, ch. 7.

15. See E. Robin, "Rapid scientific advances bring new ethical questions," *Journal of the American Medical Association* 189 (1964): 112–113; Delford L. Stickel, "Ethical and moral aspects of transplantation," *Monographs in the Surgical Sciences* 3, no. 4 (1966): 267–301; John P. Merrill, "Clinical experience is tempered by genuine human concern," *Journal of the American Medical Association* 189 (1964): 626–627; Elkington, "Moral problems in the use of borrowed organs," 189 (1964): 309–313 and "Response to moral problems of artificial and transplanted organs," 189 (1964): 363.

16. Report of the Ad Hoc Committee at Harvard Medical School to Examine the Definition of Brain Death, "A definition of irreversible coma," *Journal of the American Medical Association* 205 (1968): 337–340; Jonsen, *The Birth of Bioethics*, ch. 8.

17. "Medico-legal news" *British Medical Journal* 2 (1963): 394; "Two indicted in death of heart donor," *New York Times*, (January 28, 1969): A3.

18. "Prolongation of Life," *The Pope Speaks* 4, no. 4 (1958): 393–398.

19. *Kansas Statutes* 77-202 (Supp. 1971), quoted in the President's Commission for the Study of Ethical Problems in Medicine and Biomedical and Behavioral Research, *Defining Death: A Report on the Medical, Legal, and Ethical Issues in the Determination of Death* (Washington, D.C.: U.S. Government Printing Office, 1981), p. 62.

20. Jean Heller, "Syphilis victims in U.S. study went untreated for 40 years," *New York Times,* (July 26, 1972), A1, A8; Jonsen, *The Birth of Bioethics*, ch. 5.

21. James H. Jones, *Bad Blood* (New York: Free Press, 1981); Alan Brandt, "Racism and research: the case of the Tuskegee Study." *Hastings Center Report* 8, no. 6 (1978): 21–29; *Final Report of the Tuskegee Syphilis Study Ad Hoc Advisory Panel* (Washington, D.C.: U.S. Government Printing Office, 1973).

22. *Roe v. Wade* U.S. Supreme Court, 1973; Jonsen, *The Birth of Bioethics*, ch. 9.

23. Daniel Callahan, *Abortion: Law, Choice and Morality* (New York: Macmillan Company, 1970).

24. *In re Quinlan* New Jersey Supreme Court, 1973; Jonsen, *The Birth of Bioethics*, ch. 8.

25. Robert Edwards and Patrick Steptoe, *A Matter of Life: The Story of a Medical Breakthrough* (London: Morrow Ltd., 1980); Jonsen, *The Birth of Bioethics*, ch. 9.

26. Raymond Duff and Alastair Campbell, "Moral and ethical dilemmas in the special-

care nursery," *New England Journal of Medicine* 289 (1973): 890–894; Jonsen, *The Birth of Bioethics*, ch. 8.

27. "The Bloomington Baby," *Washington Post*, (April 18, 1982), B6; "Private death," *New York Times*, (April 27, 1982), A22.

28. George J. Annas, "The Baby Doe Regulations: governmental intervention in neonatal rescue medicine," *American Journal of Public Health* 74 (1984): 618–620. It is difficult to verify President Reagan's role in this story. The Schweiker quote in the Annas article is referenced to Norman Fost, "Putting hospitals on notice" *Hastings Center Report* 12, no. 4 (1982): 5–8, but Fost's article does not mention the president or Secretary Schweiker.

29. *Federal Register* 48 (1983), 9630–9632.

30. *Bowen v. American Hosp. Ass'n* U.S. Supreme Court, 1986.

31. *Federal Register* 50 (April 15, 1985), 14888.

32. Margery W. Shaw (ed.), *After Barney Clark. Reflections on the Utah Artificial Heart Program* (Austin: University of Texas Press, 1984); Jonsen, *The Birth of Bioethics*, ch. 7.

33. Randy Shilts, *And the Band Played On* (New York: St. Martin's Press, 1987), pp. 267, 271. Jonsen, *The Birth of Bioethics*, Epilogue.

34. Albert R. Jonsen and Jeff Stryker (eds.), *The Social Impact of AIDS in the United States* (Washington, D.C.: National Academy Press, 1993).

9. Conclusion: From Medical Ethics to Bioethics

1. Ramsey, *The Patient as Person*; Hans Jonas, "Philosophical reflections on human experimentation," *Daedalus* 98 no. 2 (1969): 219–247; Hans Jonas "Against the stream" in Hans Jonas, *Philosophical Essays: From Ancient Creed to Technological Man* (Englewood Cliffs, N.J.: Prentice-Hall, 1974); Jonsen, *The Birth of Bioethics*, chapters 2 and 3.

2. The term *bioethics* was coined by Dr. Van Rensselaer Potter in "Bioethics, the science of survival," *Perspectives in Biology and Medicine* 14 (1970): 127–153; Potter, *Bioethics: Bridge to the Future* (Englewood Cliffs, N.J.: Prentice-Hall, 1971); see Warren Reich, "The word 'bioethics': its birth and the legacies of those who shaped its meaning," *Kennedy Institute of Ethics Journal* 4 (1998): 319–336.

3. See Jonsen, *The Birth of Bioethics*, ch. 4; Tom L. Beauchamp and James F. Childress, *Principles of Biomedical Ethics* (New York: Oxford University Press, 1994).

4. Council on Ethical and Judicial Affairs, *Code of Medical Ethics. Current Opinions with Annotations* (Chicago: American Medical Association, 1998–1999).

5. Jonsen, *The Birth of Bioethics*, chapters 10 and 11.

6. David Rothman, *Strangers at the Bedside* (New York: Basic Books, 1991), pp. 189, 251.

Index

CPSIA information can be obtained
at www.ICGtesting.com
Printed in the USA
BVHW051151240622
640469BV00001B/12